# HIP-HOP NUTRITION
## VOLUME 1

## A SIMPLE, DELICIOUS, NUTRITIOUS APPROACH FOR HEALTH & FITNESS.

**James Lucas III, MS, RD, CSSD**

# CONTENTS

# TESTIMONIALS

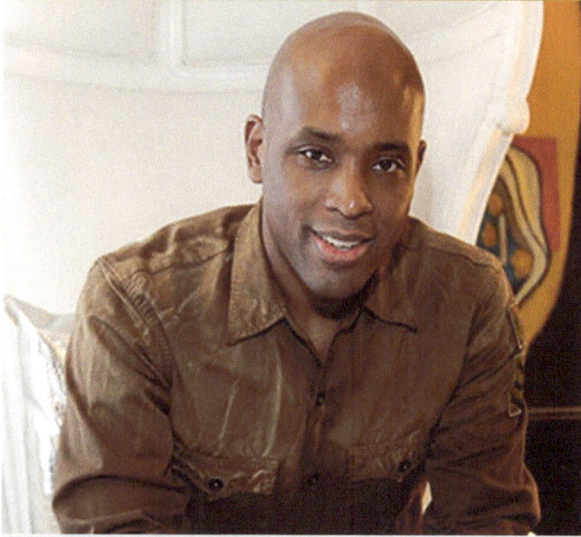

"JLucas introduced me to brussel sprouts for the first time! I never thought that I would like them, but they were absolutely delicious and according to him good for you! I recommend that any artist looking to improve health & fitness talk to JLucas Nutrition."

**DJ KELLY G.**

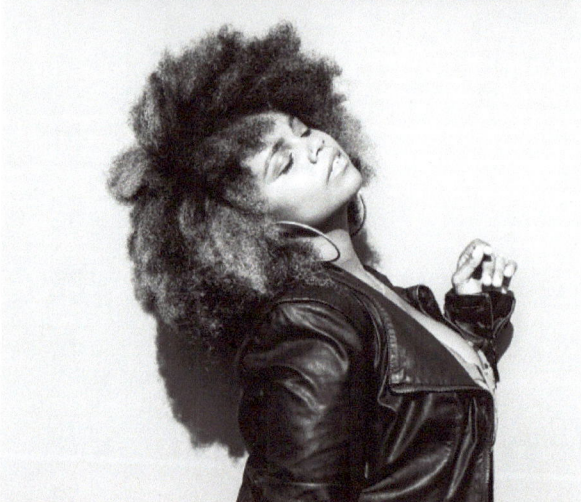

"The meal plan is working really well for me! I've never felt better in my life! You're amazing! Game changer!"

**JESSICA CHILDRESS,**
*Singer/Songwriter*

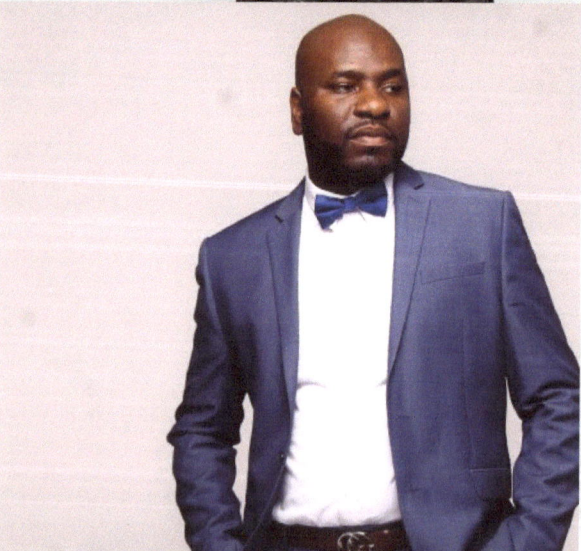

"JLucas Nutrition helped me to become more focused on my nutrition & fitness! I am eating more vegetables and recognize the importance and value of healthy eating in my life! I send all my artist to JLucas Nutrition to learn about the importance of nutrition & fitness. Use hip hop as a nutrient for your health and fitness."

**JIM-E-O,**
*My Executive Room*

# PREFACE

> "In rap music you express yourself, you tell a real story. You don't have to be politically correct! That would be wrong to hip-hop. Hip-hop is about being truthful; it's not about sparring feelings. It's about being blunt honest, harshly honest, comical, imaginative, it's about all of that, you can do what you want with rap."
>
> **NAS,** *Netflix Original Rapture.*

All my life I have been inspired by hip-hop music. I have used it as a crutch for inspiration and motivation. I love to listen to hip-hop music while working, working out or driving in the car. Hip-hop music is even what has inspired me to write this book! Let hip hop be the nutrient for your health and fitness! I hope that this book will inspire you in the same way to be passionate about your health and fitness as you are about listening to hip-hop music.

My name is James Lucas III, I was born and raised in New Haven, CT. I am a Registered Dietitian, Exercise Physiologist and Certified Specialist in Sports Dietetics (CSSD). I graduated from the University of Connecticut with a bachelor's of science in nutritional sciences and with a minor in nutrition for sport & exercise. My passion for nutrition goes back to the days when I started playing sports. I started working out at an early age, about eight years old. I had a small set of weights that my dad set up for me under his bench press. I started to learn karate when I was young and I would wear a black silk dragon printed robe ("Sho'Nuff" – The Shogun of Harlem) to school sometimes to teach my elementary school friends some karate after school.  I also didn't realize how athletic I was until in the second grade when our gym teacher had us run laps around the gym until we could not run any more.  I ran so much that I ended up being the last one still running, and my classmates cheered me on, this is when I knew I had athletic ability.

I had no idea about nutrition. Food was associated with family time and I never paid attention to what I was eating. I ate a lot of candy and would gather up some pennies from under the couch and walk across the street to our local corner store and load up on a bag of penny candies. My favorites were Sugar Daddies, Twittlerz, Laffy Taffy, potato chips, Chico sticks, you name it, and I would buy it all! My mom would make sure that my sister and I were well taken care of, providing three square meals per day. I would eat breakfast at home, the school lunch, chocolate milk and coffee cakes were my favorite and my mom would cook a good home cooked meal for dinner. I was never a picky eater and I often cleaned my plate. I even remember once spilling juice on my pancakes one Sunday morning and still finishing them off!

By the time I reached middle school I was playing football, basketball, baseball and learning Karate. My interest for being in shape and building muscle was one of my greatest concerns as a

7th grader. I would ride my bike to the local GNC store to see what kind of information the sales rep could give me about how I can build muscle, he would say "eat tuna fish," I would take that information and run with it! I remember one of my good friends that I would play with in the neighborhood would always pick on his little skinny brother. His brother wanted to build muscle so I told him "eat tuna fish!" This is where my first set of nutrition recommendations started, but I was a long way from knowing that I would become a Registered Dietitian.

For those who may not know, Registered Dietitians (RDs) are the food and nutrition experts who can translate the science of nutrition into practical solutions for healthy living. RDs use their nutrition expertise to help individuals make unique, positive lifestyle changes. They work in the community, hospitals, schools, public health clinics, nursing homes, fitness centers, food management, food industry, universities, research and private practice settings. RDs are advocates for advancing the nutritional status of Americans and people around the world. Hip-Hop Nutrition: Volume 1 is my unique way to encourage, teach and empower you to make positive lifestyle changes that will last a lifetime.

Oftentimes we just eat, not thinking about how the food choices we make can have a cumulative, long-term effect on our health, wellness and risk for chronic diseases. Do you ever think about how food can affect your health and wellness? This book is designed to create a paradigm shift in the way you think about food. I will be providing you with information about nutrition and food to help you to eat healthier. The principles that I will provide you with can be applied to anyone, whether you are sedentary, active or an athlete. I know that nutrition can be complicated and many don't know what to eat. We are also surround by lots of yummy, unhealthy delicious foods which makes it hard for us to make consistent healthy choices.

This is a simple, delicious and nutritious recipe book that will be easy to follow for real results! This book will provide you with the principles necessary to help you to improve your health support your weight loss effort, help you to build more muscle or to keep you in shape. I would like you to allow this recipe book to shift in your thinking around food and nutrition to help you optimize on your health, wellness and daily performance. Hip-Hop Nutrition: Volume 1 will make you a smarter food consumer to help you recognize the influence of the foods you eat on your health. This book is designed to empower you to have the basic nutritional tools you need to create well balanced meals for health and fitness. You don't have to be a chef to know how to cook healthy meals. This book contains 21 simple, delicious and nutritious hip-hop inspired, recipes for your health and fitness! You can select a recipe for breakfast, lunch or dinner seven days a week for a meal plan that you can use for a lifetime! Health is wealth! Invest in yourself! Start reading and following these recipes today to start seeing your full genetic potential for health, wellness and fitness!

# ACKNOWLEDGMENTS

Your only as strong as your weakest link. It takes unity to create power. You need daily energy, but your bandwidth can only take you so far, that's what a team is important to help you build an empire. I would like to acknowledge and thank the following individuals for supporting this project:

| | |
|---|---|
| JOSE LOPEZ | AMENA ZENO |
| CYDNEY SWEENEY | JESSICA M. |
| KEVIN SAINT CLAIR | LA'ERICA WILLIAMS |
| CYNTHIA WATSON | MICHAEL BUAN |
| RAQUEL REYES | THOMAS FEDOCK |
| BRAD TOWNSEND | JAMIE GREER |
| JESSICA CHILDRESS | TYRONE WASHINGTON |
| TIMOTHY MONK | AL WASHINGTON |
| MATT MORAN | DWIGHT CLEMMONS |
| OMAR KINNEBREW | JESSE PHILLIPS |
| MICAEL GEORGE | FELICIA LANIER |
| CARMEN ORDONEZ | MAURICE WATSON |
| RICHARD MUTTS | RICHARD JAGGERS |
| PATRICIA DIXON | OMAR BROWN |
| ALEXANDER SMITH | SONIA SIMS |
| LARA GHAZOUL | MICHAEL SHAOLIAN |
| LAPRAYA LITTLE | AERON MARVEL |

# INTRODUCTION

"It's 2:30 and the sun is beaming air conditioner broke, and I hear my stomach screaming; Hungry for anything unhealthy and if nutrition can help me I'll tell you to suck my %$! @, then I'll continue eating"

**K. LAMAR** *The Art of Peer Pressure*

In the hip-hop world we tend to eat anything without thinking about how it may affect our health. Fried chicken, biscuits, gravy, macaroni and cheese, French fries, hamburgers, potato chips, honey buns, soda, and cake just to name a few. It's not that these foods can't fit into a healthy diet, because believe me even I like to indulge in these foods too, but what's important is choosing these foods in moderation and more importantly including plenty of fruits and vegetables throughout the day. For instance, how many fruits and vegetables did you have today? How about yesterday? This is where we should have a majority of our focus when it comes to eating, making the foundation of meals rich in fruits and vegetables, because currently there is a major discrepancy between the amount of unhealthy foods we choose to eat and the proportion of fruits and vegetables we consume daily. Increasing your fruit and vegetable intake is a major key to reducing the risk for disease and increasing your life span.

Did you know that the top five chronic diseases are related to diet (Eatright.org: Journal of The Academy of Nutrition and Dietetics)? Risk factors for chronic disease begin early in life, but evidence shows that making dietary and lifestyle changes may prevent the development and progression of disease and help to reduce the risk for premature death. Here are the top "preventable" chronic diseases:

1. **HEART DISEASE & STROKE** – The leading cause of death in the U.S. for 100+ years and currently accounts for 1 in 3 deaths. Stroke 1 in 18 deaths in the U.S.

2. **OBESITY** – 1 in 3 adults in the U.S. is obese. Obesity in all age, ethnic and gender groups within the U.S. has reached epidemic proportions.

3. **CANCER** – claims more lives than heart disease among people younger than 85 years of age. Causing factors: Obesity (preventable), poor diet, physical inactivity (preventable). Following a low fat diet with 30% of calories or less coming from fat can be effective in reducing risk of breast cancer and ovarian cancers. Moderate to vigorous exercise results in 30% reduction of colon cancer risk.

4. **OSTEOPOROSIS** – 8% of 20+ year old females in the U.S. are affected Bone fracture prevention is strongly linked to weight-bearing exercise and vitamin D and calcium intake.

5. **DIABETES** – 18+ million U.S. adults diagnosed with type 2 diabetes in 2008. Diabetes prevalence is projected to reach 33% by 2050. 12.7% of 12-19-year olds have metabolic syndrome which predisposes them to risk of type 2 diabetes in young adulthood and beyond. Predictors of type 2 diabetes: obesity, family history, high triglyceride levels, high blood pressure, low high-density (HDL) cholesterol.

This recipe book is designed to act as a guide to provide you with some healthier alternatives to the more "unhealthy" traditional dishes that we are accustom to in hip-hop culture. Let's better ourselves and make more of a conscious effort to be healthy and live healthier! For health, wealth, and prosperity!

The calorie and nutrition information provided with each recipe represent approximate values. You may modify each recipe according to your liking. I would recommend sticking with the foundation of the recipe; however, you may change certain ingredients if you have a food preference, food dislike, intolerance, or allergy. The recipes are not designed to induce weight loss, but rather provide a healthier alternative to more commonly eaten unhealthy foods. You have a greater probability of improving your health and potentially inducing weight loss by following portion control, including more fruits and vegetables and by committing to a daily exercise routine. You can mix and match recipes and select the meal of choice for breakfast, lunch, or dinner. Remember to include low calorie, sugar free beverages with meals and be mindful of the number of calories you may be consuming from juice, sodas, and alcohol.

The average total calories per day for each recipe when combining breakfast, lunch, and dinner would be approximately 1500 calories, 115 g protein, 113 g carbohydrate and 62g fat which is about 31% protein, 30% carbohydrate and 39% fat per day. This ratio will change according to the serving size you select for each meal in addition to beverages and snacks that you may add with or between meals. I would not focus so much on the numbers, but rather look at the portion size, food choices, non-starchy vegetable intake and distribution of food throughout the day. If your goal is weight loss, then it would be important to eat less food and move more. If you are looking to build muscle, maintain weight or you are highly physically active then you should consider doubling up on the portion sizes for each recipe. Here are a few quick tips and ideas to further support your health, wellness, and fitness needs:

## Curb your appetite and muscle up with lean protein!

These artist have it right when referring to protein to get in shape and lose weight. Increasing your protein intake is just as important as adequate fruits and vegetables when observing the benefits

"I'm back in shape, Pour Crystal in the blender and make a protein shake!"

**50 CENT,** Hustler's Ambition

3

for supporting weight loss, muscle building or maintenance. Protein is a major nutrient for supporting a healthy diet. Proteins are made up of amino acids, the building blocks for enzymes, hormones, vitamins, bones, muscles, cartilage, skin, and blood. Protein foods can be found in both animal (i.e. meats, chicken, fish, eggs, and diary) or plant base foods (i.e. soy, legumes, nuts, seeds, grains, some vegetables, and fruits). You should aim for 25 - 35 grams of protein per meal depending on your activity level and age. Older adults have higher protein needs than younger individuals because they have a more difficult time utilizing protein, so more is needed to maintain and build muscle mass. High protein diets have been associated with supporting weight loss, and building and maintaining muscle mass. A lean protein diet helps to keep you full, improves appetite, controls hunger, and helps to preserve muscle mass for the active or aging individual. You lose 8% of your muscle per decade after the age of 40 and 15% after the age of 70. Eating a high protein diet and including weight training can help reduce the loss of muscle over time. Animal based protein foods also contain B vitamins such as niacin, thiamin, riboflavin, B6 and B12, vitamin E, iron, zinc, and magnesium to support energy and bodily functions. Your protein needs will generally be met a little easier with an animal-based protein rich diet, however if you are following a plant-based diet you can certainly meet your protein needs by choosing higher protein plant base foods like pea, soy, hemp, quinoa, rice, beans, and seeds.

Here is a reference from 2017 International Society of Sports Nutrition Position Stand on Protein and Exercise:

- Aim to evenly distribute your protein intake throughout the day (i.e. 20-40 g protein per meal) every 3-4 hours.

- If you are an athlete or highly active person currently attempting to lose body fat while preserving lean muscle mass, a daily intake of 1.5-2.2g/kg bodyweight (0.68-1g/lb bodyweight) would be a good target. For example an 180 lb person (81.8kg) would need to consume 123 – 180 grams of protein per day.

- If you are an athlete or highly active person, or you are attempting to lose body fat while preserving lean mass, then a daily intake of 1.0-1.5g/kg bodyweight (0.45-0.68g/lb bodyweight) would be a good target. For example an 180 lb person (81.8kg) would need to consume 82 – 123g protein per day.

- If you are sedentary and not looking to change body composition, a daily target of 0.8g/kg bodyweight (0.36g/lb bodyweight) and upwards would be a good target. For example an 180 lb person (81.8kg) would need to consume 66g protein per day

- For building muscle mass and for maintaining muscle mass through a positive muscle protein balance, an overall daily protein intake in the range of 1.4-2.0 g protein/kg body weight/ day (g/kg/d) is sufficient for most exercising individuals, a value that falls in line within the Acceptable Macronutrient Distribution Range published by the Institute of Medicine for protein. For example an 180 lb person (81.8kg) would need to consume 115 - 164g protein per day

- Don't be afraid to take in super high amounts of protein (if you have normal kidney function)! There is novel evidence that suggests higher protein intakes (>3.0 g/kg/d) may have positive effects on body composition in resistance-trained individuals (i.e. promote loss of fat mass). For example an 180 lb person (81.8kg) would need to consume 245 g or more of protein per day.

- If you are obese (BMI greater than 30 or body fat over 20% for males and 30% for females) then consider calculating your needs based upon your target weight. For example if you weigh 300 lb (136.36 kg) and calculated your protein needs for weight loss at 2g/kg, then your needs would be 273g protein per day (1090 calories from protein). Rather use a realistic goal weight 200 lbs and calculate your protein needs for a 200 lb individual (90.9 kg) at 2g/kg body weight for 182 grams protein per day (728 calories)

If you are confused as to which of the above needs would be appropriate for you then reach out to you local Registered Dietitian for more specifics.

## Use the Plate Method

This is one of the simplest, most effective, principles that you can apply to your diet for simple, real, results! At each meal focus on covering half your plate with one cup of non-starchy

- Artichoke
- Asparagus
- Beets
- Broccoli
- Brussels sprouts
- Cabbage
- Carrots

- Cauliflower
- Celery
- Cucumber
- Eggplant
- Green onions
- Kale
- Lettuce

- Mushrooms
- Okra
- Peppers, all varieties
- Spinach
- Tomato
- Summer Squash
- Zucchini

FILL HALF OF A 9-INCH PLATE WITH ONE CUP OF NON-STARCHY VEGETABLES, A QUATER OF THE PLATE WITH HIGH-PROTEIN FOODS, AND A QUARTER PLATE WITH CARBOHYDRATE FOODS. ADD A SMALL SERING OF FRUIT & A SERVING OF DAIRY.

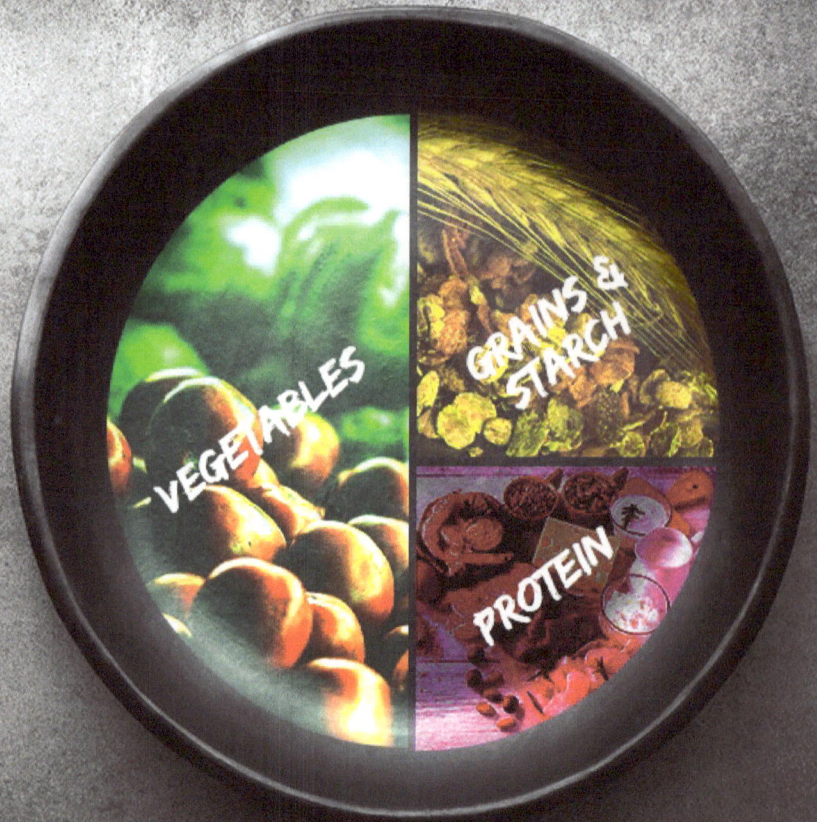

vegetables; a quarter of the plate with high-protein lean foods; and a quarter of the plate with carbohydrates. Too often we see the opposite ratio of one quarter to no quarter vegetables with half the plate covered with carbohydrates(i.e. rice) and the remaining portion filled with protein. Here is a list of non-starchy vegetables to fill half your plate with:

## Be mindful of how much you "drank"

If you "drank" too much alcohol it can derail your health, fitness, and wellness plan. Alcohol in moderation is key. Moderate is defined as approximately 1-2 drinks per day for women and men, respectively. An alcoholic drink is defined as 12 oz. (355 mL) of 5% beer, 5 oz. (150 mL) 12.5% wine, or 1.5 oz. (45 mL) of drinks with a higher (40%) alcohol content.

"Pour up, drank, head shot, drank, sit down, drank, stand up, drank, pass out, drank, wake up, drank, faded, drank, faded, drank..."

**KENDRICK LAMAR,**
Swimming Pools (Drank)

We should recognize that alcohol takes precedence on metabolism when ingested. Meaning the body will focus on breaking down alcohol before fats, carbohydrates, or protein because alcohol is essentially a toxin, so the body is focusing on stabilizing alcohol so that it does not poison us. If you are aiming for weight loss and are consuming too much alcohol daily, then it will make weight loss that much harder. Think about your fat burning ability being shut off with each sip of alcohol. If you're aiming for weight loss cutting back on alcohol intake may be a good start!

Additionally, for juices be mindful of how much juice you are drinking. I personally do not drink much juice at all. Think about an orange if you were to squeeze it for fresh juice it would probably only provide a quarter of the typical juice that you would poor in a glass. A glass of orange juice may be equal to 5-6 freshly squeezed oranges. Cut the juice in half by diluting with water.

## Healthy Snacks

For the more common unhealthy snacks that you may prefer it might be easier to avoid eating them if you keep them out of your sight. Use the principle "out of sight, out of mind" to reduce cravings for empty calorie foods like chips, cakes, pies, and candy. You don't always have to snack in between meals, but rather check your appetite to see if adding a snack may be necessary. Also, consider how long it may be before your next meal. If you have any more than two hours before your next meal and your appetite is between 5-10 on a scale of 1 least hungry to 10 most hunger then I would say consume a small healthy snack to help reduce cravings for empty calorie junk foods, in addition may help with portion control during meal times.

Here are a list of snacks that you can consider to help keep your health and appetite in check!
- Nuts (i.e. ¼ c almonds, cashews, peanuts, pecans, walnuts)
- Dark chocolate (1 oz. of 70% cocoa or greater, helps to reduce craving for other sweets!)
- Protein bars (Aim for at least 20 g of protein per serving)
- Ready to drink protein shakes (Aim for at least 15g of protein per serving)
- Greek yogurt
- Dried fruit (i.e. ¼ c raisins, apricots, apples, peaches)
- Whole fruits (i.e. 1 apple, 1 orange, 1 peach, 1 plum, 1 pear, 1 cup of pineapples or watermelon)
- Vegetables (i.e. 1 cup of carrot sticks, broccoli, peppers, beets)
- Beef Jerky
- Cheese stick (1 oz.)

## Keep the carbs in check!

We have a significantly high presence of carbohydrate foods in our diet. Carbohydrate foods provide the fuel we need for the brain and working muscles, which makes them more important for athletes. We do have a limit to how much carbohydrates can be store in the muscle tissue, so it is important to be mindful of your total calorie intake as to not overindulge. Additionally, we want to aim for the more wholesome carbohydrates that will come from fruits and starches such as potatoes, beans, and grains. These foods will provide more nutrients and especially fiber which is important for managing blood sugars, supporting digestive health, and keeping you full. Today, we have an overabundance of processed carbohydrate foods. Focus on this component of your diet more than anything else because of the high probability of eating more carbohydrates than your body needs, unless you are an athlete or highly active. Keep the following refined, processed carbohydrates in check, before you wreck yourself!

- Cereals
- Breads
- Crackers
- Cakes
- Pasta
- Rice
- Tortillas
- French Fries
- Chips
- Soda
- Juices
- Popcorn
- Candy
- Waffles
- Bagels
- Donuts

## Recipe Tips:

Read the recipe completely before you start making it to be sure you understand the process.

Check to make sure that you have all ingredients prior to making the recipe. Make twice the amount of the recipe to use later in the week.

Make a grocery list and stick to it! Make sure you eat a snack prior to grocery shopping to reduce the chances that you will purchase foods or items not on your list.

Use frozen or precut vegetables, pre-chopped garlic (in a jar in the produce section of the market), dried onions instead of fresh, etc. You can make the recipes with whole, fresh ingredients if you prefer, but the goal is to make the recipes simple.

Use the metric conversions chart in the appendix for continental cooking.

You can add, modify, and customize each recipe according to your preference. For instance, it may be best to add a protein food to your oatmeal such as eggs; you can choose to make whole eggs or egg whites. You may also consider making each meal vegetarian by eliminating the meats, chicken or fish.

For those with hypertension consider using a salt substitute or cutting the salt intake in half for each recipe.

Check out all 21 simple, delicious and nutritious recipes in this book to discover which ones are your favorites. You can follow a different recipe each day for breakfast, lunch and dinner for a seven day meal plan; or you can choose the same recipes for breakfast, lunch and dinner every day to start seeing simple, real, results for health and fitness!

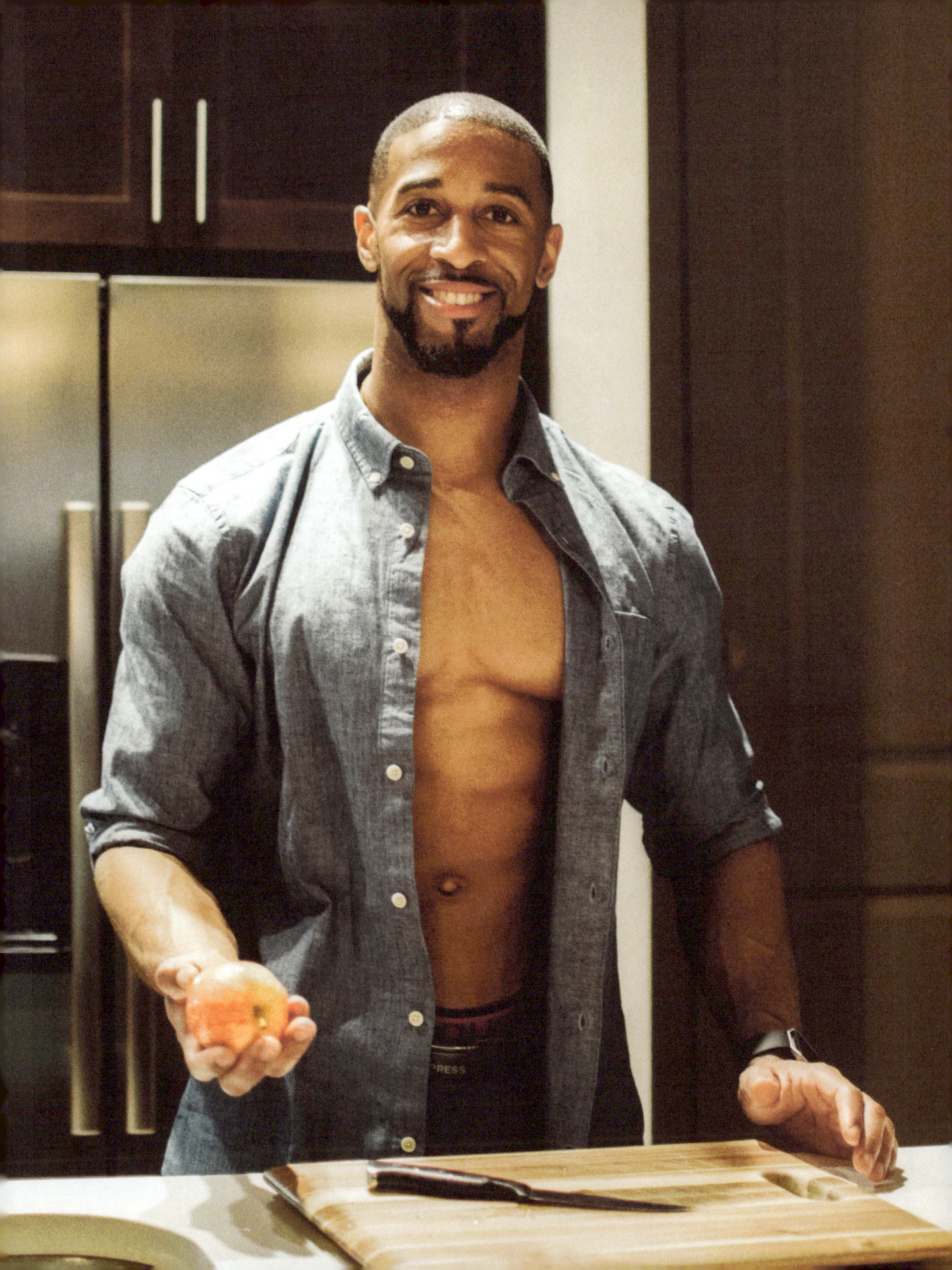

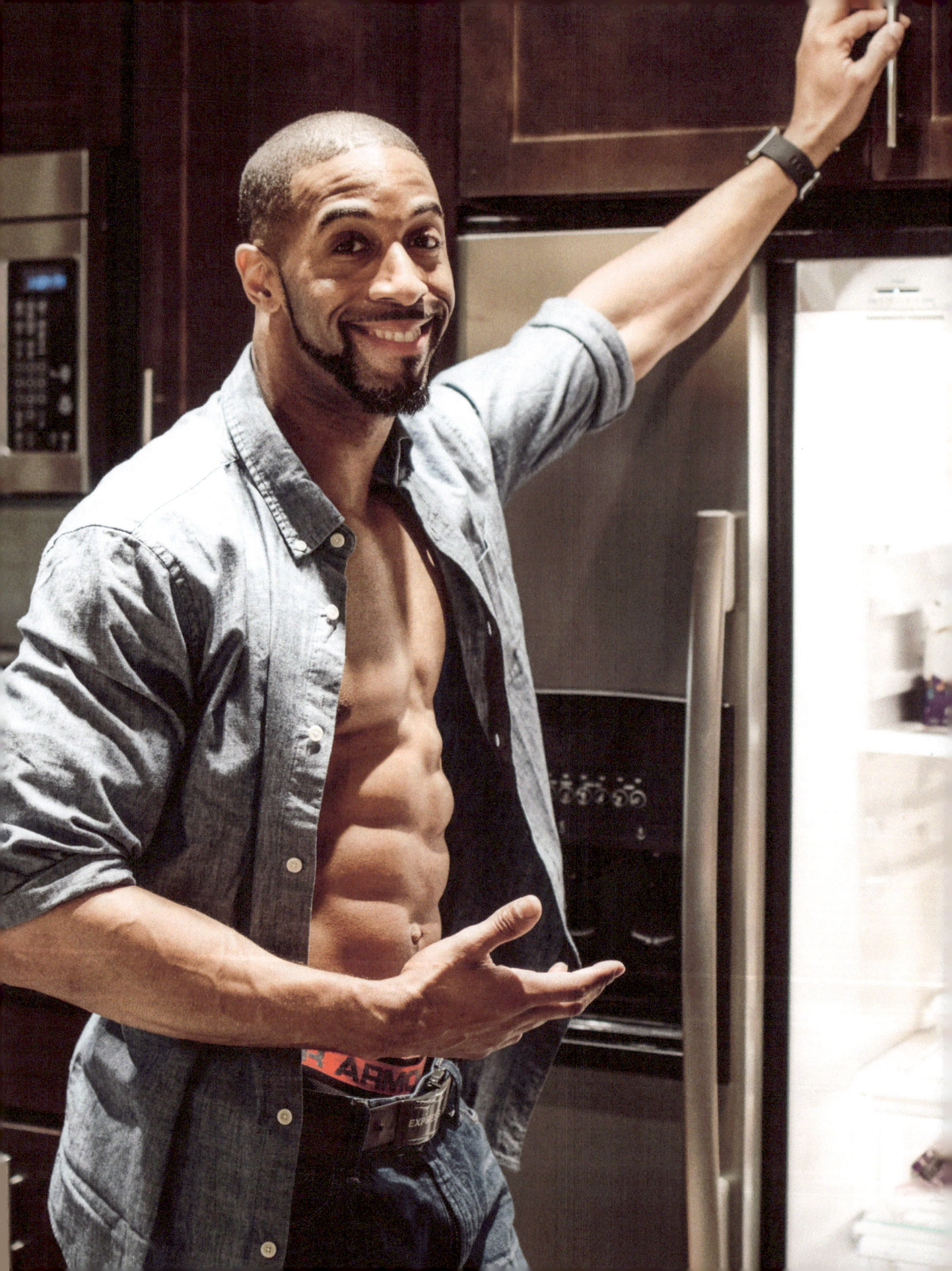

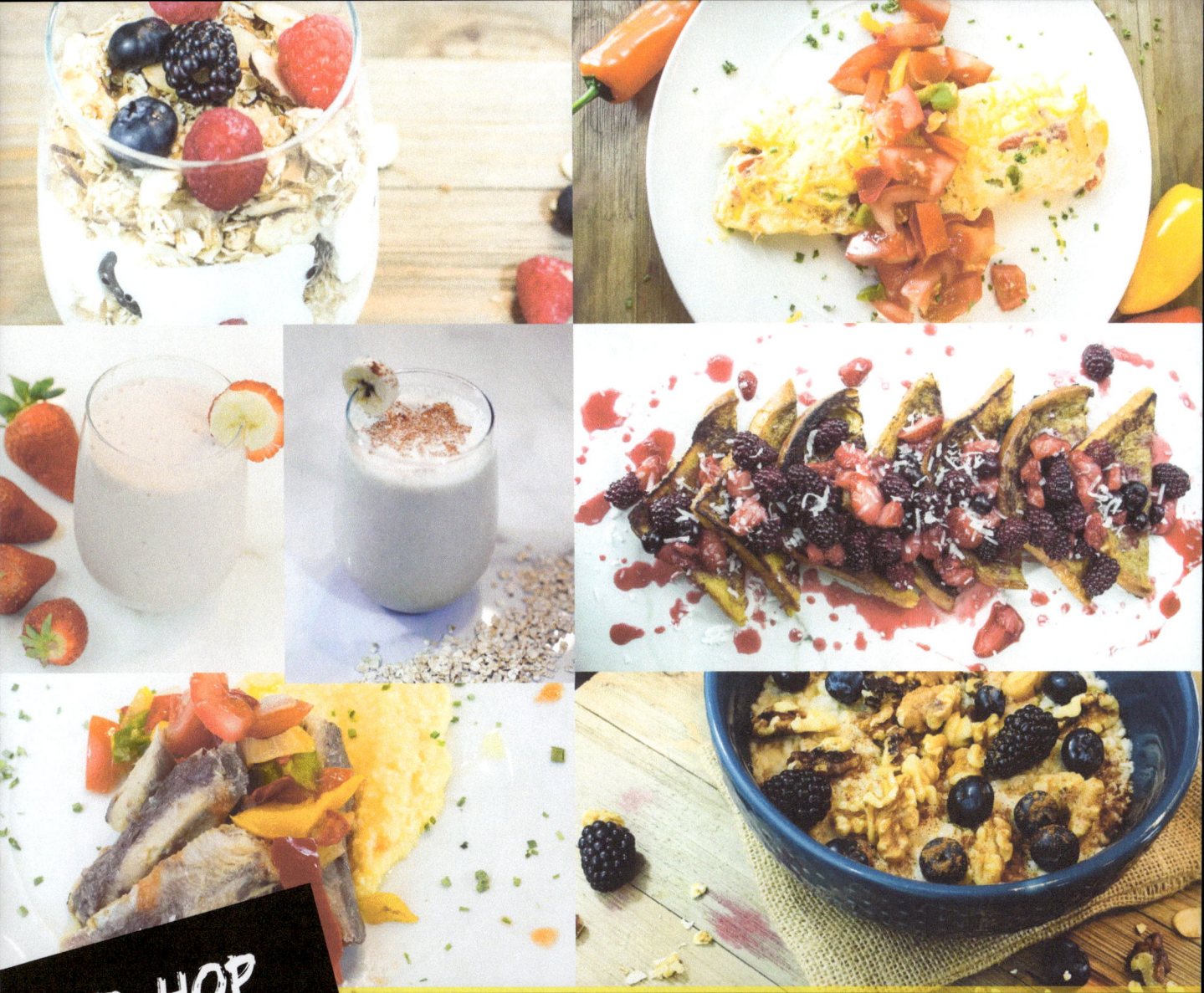

# HIP-HOP HEALTHY BREAKFAST RECIPES

Breakfast is often noted as the most important meal of the day. If you are accustom to eating breakfast every day you should continue to do so to support your daily nutritional intake. However, not everyone eats breakfast every day. I would encourage breakfast as it as another opportunity for you to increase your fruit and vegetable intake, which has a major role in reducing your overall risk for disease. Particularly, if you have diabetes breakfast becomes much more important for glycemic control. During breakfast you should focus on protein as the staple of the meal, while keeping total carbohydrates below 30-45 grams, include at least one serving of fruit or vegetables. Cereal is a common stable of many breakfast dishes, but they are often high in sugar. Check out the nutrition facts label for the total amount of carbohydrates per serving, they should be below 30g per servings. Start following the JLucas Nutrition Hip-Hop Breakfast recipes for a simple, delicious and nutritious breakfast that will be high in protein, low in fat, rich in fiber and disease fighting fruits and vegetables for health and fitness.

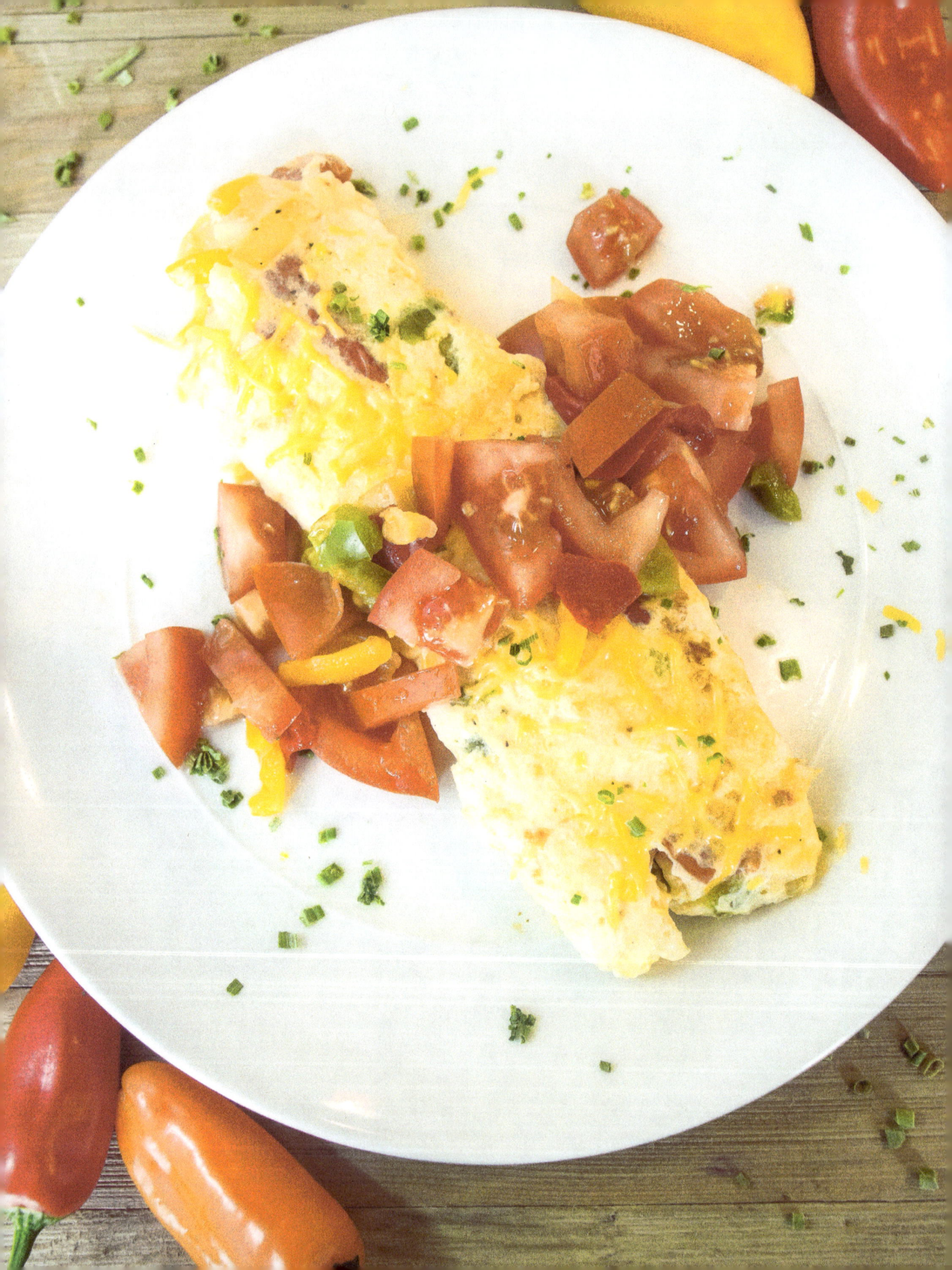

# "GOOD MORNING" VEGETABLES & EGGS - WHOLE

## Ingredients:

- 2 large whole eggs or 1 cup pasteurized egg whites
- 1 cup non-starchy vegetables
- (i.e. spinach or peppers or onions or tomatoes or chopped broccoli)
- 1 tbsp. olive oil
- ½ teaspoon salt
- Dash of pepper
- Optional: 1 oz. low fat cheddar or Colby cheese

This recipe calls for whole eggs and vegetables for a protein filled meal to keep you full throughout the day. Eggs have received a bad rap in the past, "I don't eat my green eggs and ham", however they are very nutritious and delicious! Eggs provide 6 grams of high-quality protein per serving for mental and physical energy; they are very cost effective at approximately 17 cents per serving; the yolks provide choline to promote normal cell activity, liver function and the transport of nutrients through the body. It also contains an anti-oxidant known as lutein which helps to protect eye health. Add vegetables to your eggs for a healthy, hearty dish! You can add 1-2 egg whites and cheese for some additional protein to help keep you full and to support muscle tissue for physical activity or weight loss! The good morning egg white version is a way to cut back on the calories, fat and cholesterol if you have a history of heart disease or are aiming for weight loss. Both the whole eggs and egg whites can fit into a healthy diet, especially in moderation. Alternate between the whole egg and the egg white recipe throughout the week to help meet your protein needs during breakfast!

## Directions:

1. Heat non-stick skillet on medium heat,
2. Heat olive oil simultaneously
3. Add vegetables and cook for 5 min
4. Add eggs to skillet and scramble
5. Add salt and pepper to taste and serve!

## Nutrition Facts

1 servings per container

**Serving size**

| | |
|---|---|
| **Amount Per Serving** | |
| **Calories** | **360** |

| | % Daily Value* |
|---|---|
| **Total Fat** 24g | **31%** |
| Saturated Fat 5g | 25% |
| *Trans* Fat 0g | |
| **Cholesterol** 355mg | **118%** |
| **Sodium** 1540mg | **67%** |
| **Total Carbohydrate** 11g | **4%** |
| Dietary Fiber 3g | 11% |
| Total Sugars 0g | |
| Includes 0g Added Sugars | 0% |
| **Protein** 20g | **40%** |

Not a significant source of vitamin D, calcium, iron, and potassium

\* The % Daily Value (DV) tells you how much a nutrient in a serving of food contributes to a daily diet. 2,000 calories a day is used for general nutrition advice.

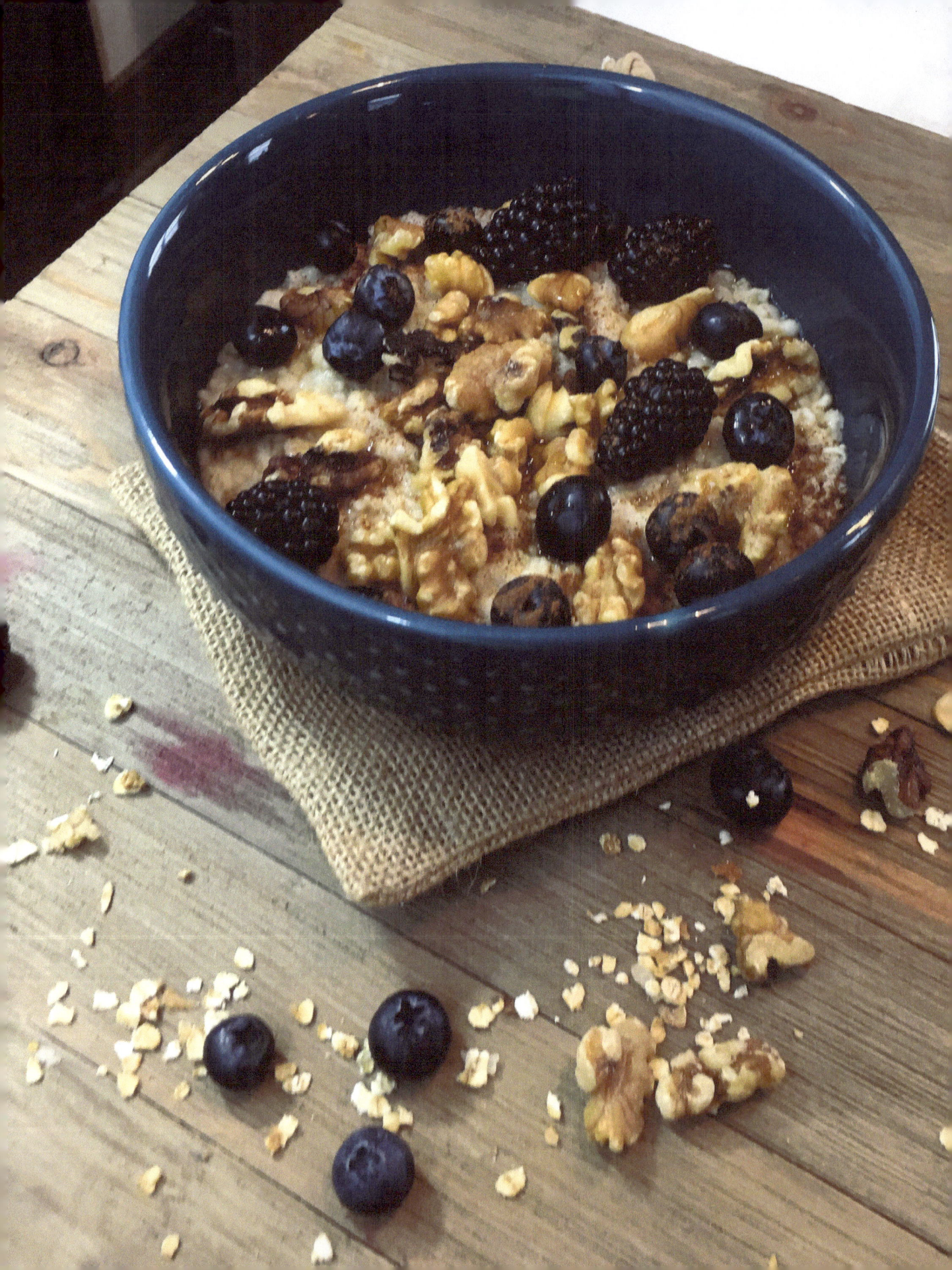

# LIL "LOADED" OATMEAL

## Ingredients:

- ½ cup -Quick 1-Minute Oats
- 1 cup water
- 1 tablespoon walnuts or almonds
- ½ cup black berries or blueberries or raspberries
- 2 oz. unsweetened vanilla almond milk
- Dash cinnamon
- Optional: 1 tablespoon shredded coconut

Oatmeal is a great staple of any breakfast dish. It is rich in soluble fiber which helps to reduce cholesterol. The key with oatmeal is to implement portion control. Measure out your portions or use packets of unsweetened oatmeal to keep sugar and calorie intake under control. This recipe is made from the Quaker Oats Quick Oats and allows you to add healthy ingredients such as walnuts and berries. Allow the fruit to flavor your oatmeal, but if you're tempted to go sweeter make sure to use moderation. Add eggs or make a protein shake to increase the protein content of your oatmeal. Load it up, toss it up and enjoy!

## Directions (Makes One Serving):

1. Add ½ cup of quick oats to a bowl
2. Add 1 cup of water and mix
3. Place in microwave for 1 minute
4. Remove from microwave and add nuts, fruit and toppings of choice and enjoy!

## Nutrition Facts

1 servings per container

| Serving size | 1 |
|---|---|

**Amount Per Serving**

| Calories | 350 |
|---|---|

% Daily Value*

| | |
|---|---|
| **Total Fat** 11g | 14% |
| Saturated Fat 1g | 5% |
| *Trans* Fat 0g | |
| **Cholesterol** 0mg | 0% |
| **Sodium** 60mg | 3% |
| **Total Carbohydrate** 59g | 21% |
| Dietary Fiber 6g | 21% |
| Total Sugars 0g | |
| Includes 0g Added Sugars | 0% |
| **Protein** 8g | 16% |

Not a significant source of vitamin D, calcium, iron, and potassium

*The % Daily Value (DV) tells you how much a nutrient in a serving of food contributes to a daily diet. 2,000 calories a day is used for general nutrition advice.

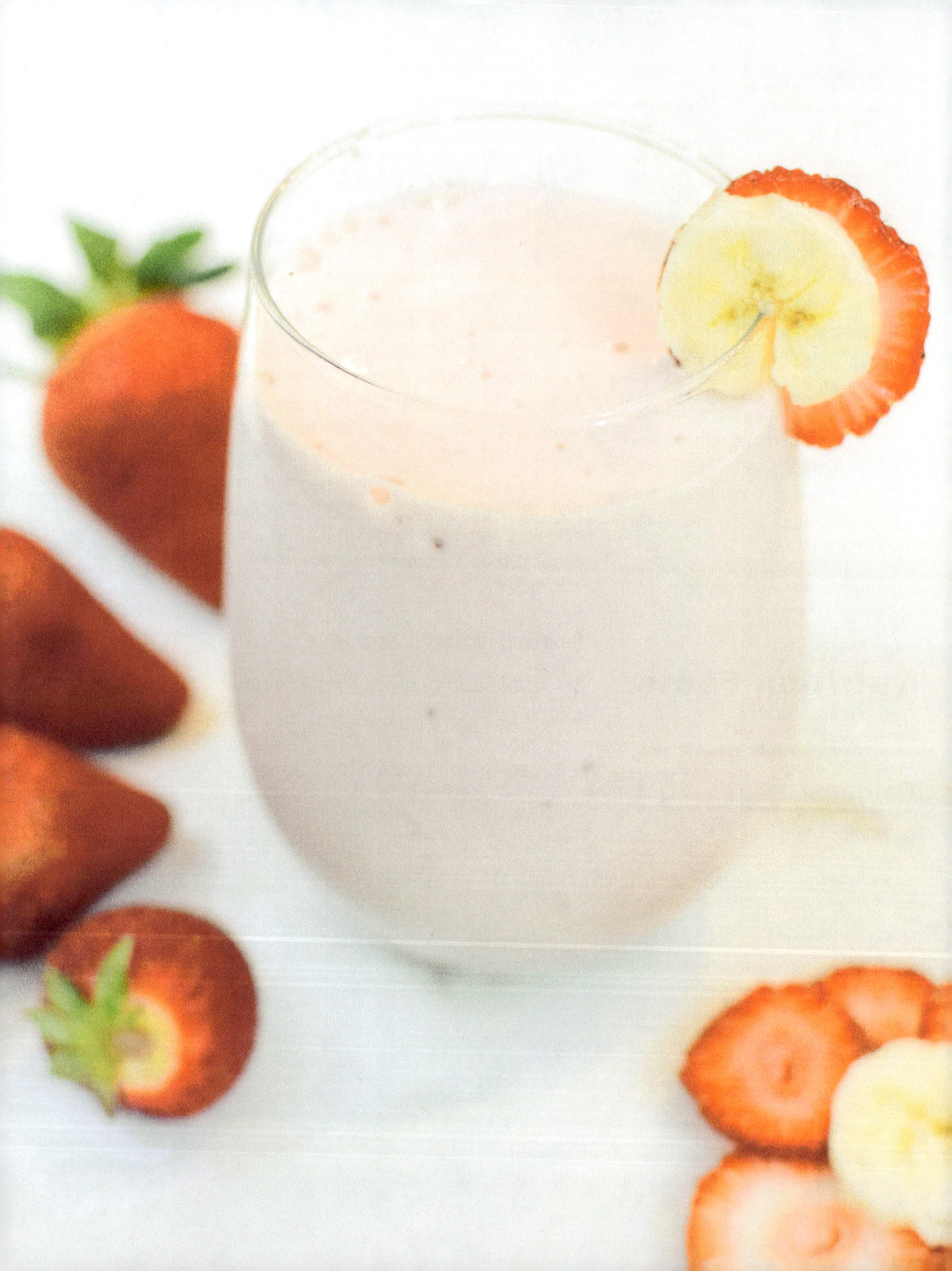

# FABULICIOUS STRAWBERRY BANANA PROTEIN SHAKE

Protein shakes can be a quick, simple, delicious, and nutritious option to make and take on the go! This Fabulous shake is made with four ingredients. Throw them in the blender and be on your way to better health, wellness, and fitness. You could consider drinking this protein shake after a workout. The psyllium is an option to add to your shake. It will make the protein shake thicker and provide additional soluble fiber to keep you full and fit!

## Ingredients:

- 8 oz. almond milk or skim milk or coconut milk or rice milk or almond milk
- 1 scoop of whey protein
- 1 cup fresh or frozen strawberries
- ½ banana
- Optional: 1 tablespoon psyllium fiber

## Directions:

1. Use your blender to create this recipe.

2. Add 8 oz. of the milk of your choice then the remaining ingredients.

3. Blend for 60 seconds and enjoy!

## Nutrition Facts

1 servings per container

**Serving size** 1

**Amount Per Serving**

**Calories** 280

| | % Daily Value* |
|---|---|
| **Total Fat** 5g | 6% |
| Saturated Fat 1g | 5% |
| *Trans* Fat 0g | |
| **Cholesterol** 65mg | 22% |
| **Sodium** 240mg | 10% |
| **Total Carbohydrate** 35g | 13% |
| Dietary Fiber 11g | 39% |
| Total Sugars 0g | |
| Includes 0g Added Sugars | 0% |
| **Protein** 25g | 50% |

Not a significant source of vitamin D, calcium, iron, and potassium

*The % Daily Value (DV) tells you how much a nutrient in a serving of food contributes to a daily diet. 2,000 calories a day is used for general nutrition advice.

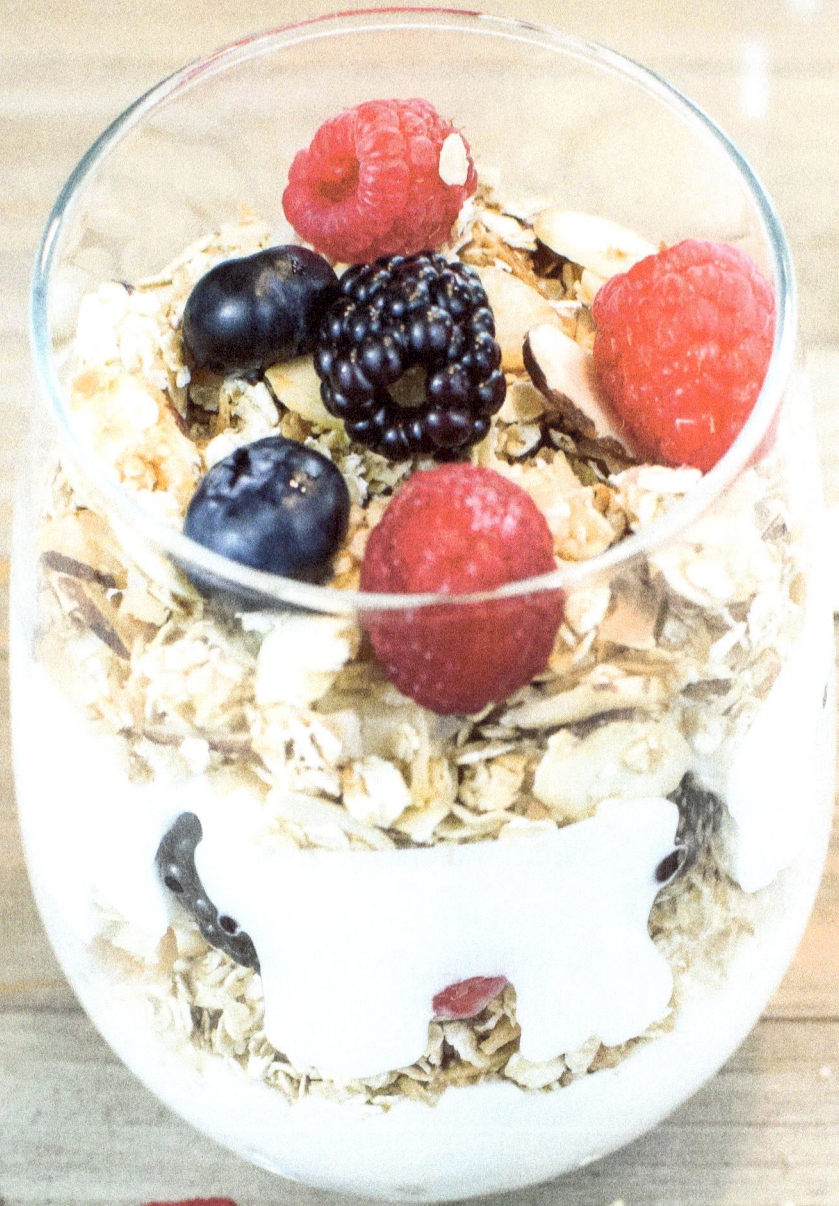

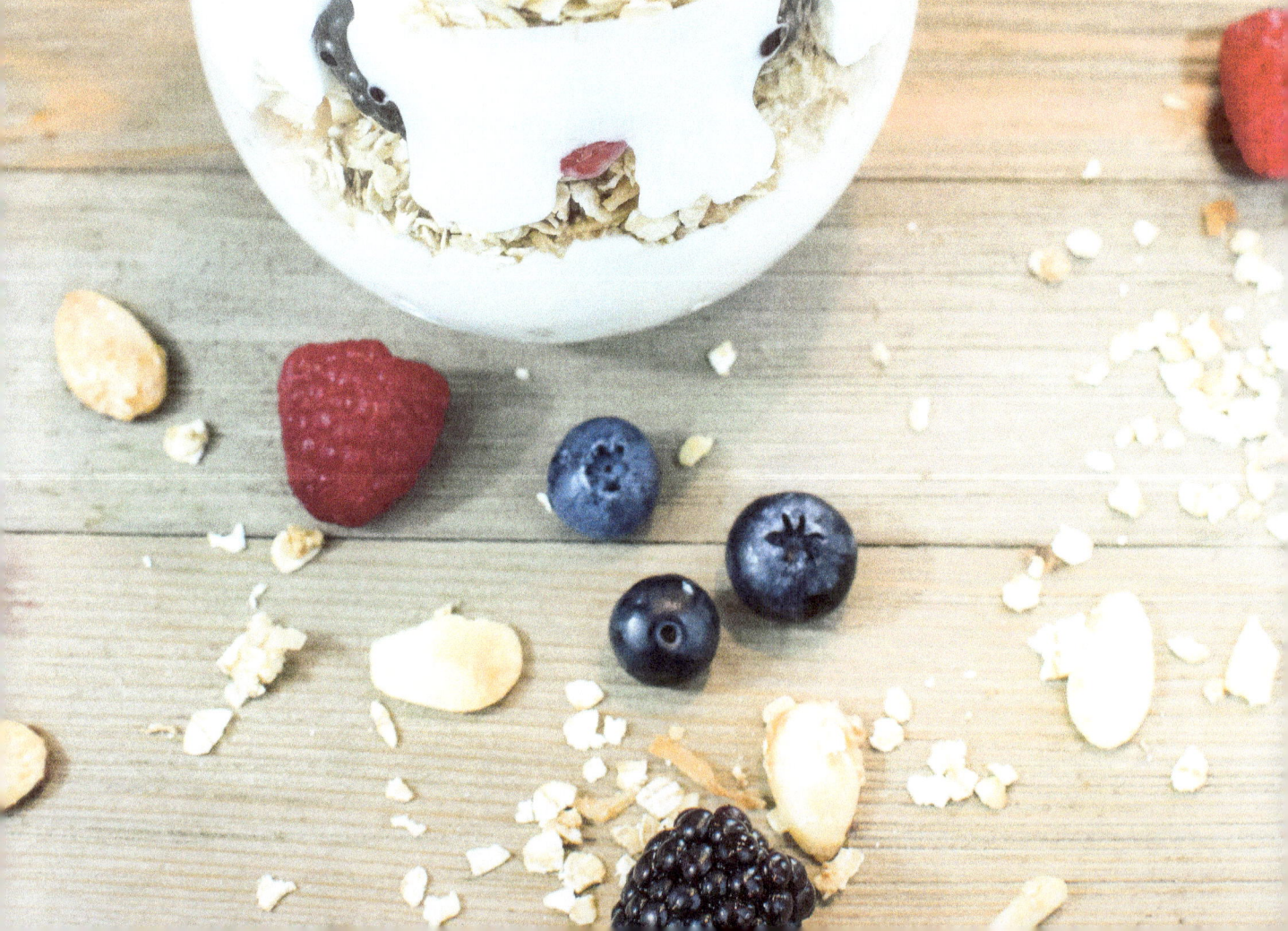

# WELL YA KNOWYA GRONOLYA

## Ingredients:

- 1 cup of Oats
- ¼ cup nuts chopped (almonds, pecans, walnuts)
- 2 teaspoon vanilla extract
- 2 tablespoons of honey
- 2 tablespoon canola oil or coconut oil
- ½ teaspoon salt
- Dash of cinnamon (optional)
- ¼ cup shredded coconut flakes (optional)

Cereal is very common as a breakfast option. If you look in most people's cabinets, you will find a box of cereal or two…or three. Cereals can be healthy, but they can also be empty and full of sugar. They key is to choose a high fiber cereal with little (less than 3-5g) of added sugar and to add some fruit to it such as sliced bananas or blueberries. This granola is a very cost effective healthy way to make your own cereal that you can pour a glass of milk over or bag it up and take with you on the go for a snack. Goes well with Greek yogurt. Try it with eggs on the side or a protein shake, and I know you'll clap!

## Directions:

1. Preheat the oven to 300ºF

2. Combine all ingredients in a large mixing bowl. Mix well and toss.

3. Spread the mixture in a thin layer on a baking sheet lined with paper parchment and bake for 10 minutes until lightly toasted.

4. Cool and store in a large zip lock bag or airtight container. Add to Greek yogurt or eat a handful between meals as a snack!

## Nutrition Facts

4 servings per container

| Serving size | 1/4 cup |
|---|---|

**Amount Per Serving**

| Calories | 210 |
|---|---|

| | % Daily Value* |
|---|---|
| **Total Fat** 11g | **14%** |
| Saturated Fat 1g | **5%** |
| *Trans* Fat 0g | |
| **Cholesterol** 0mg | **0%** |
| **Sodium** 290mg | **13%** |
| **Total Carbohydrate** 24g | **9%** |
| Dietary Fiber 3g | **11%** |
| Total Sugars 0g | |
| Includes 0g Added Sugars | **0%** |
| **Protein** 4g | **8%** |

Not a significant source of vitamin D, calcium, iron, and potassium

*The % Daily Value (DV) tells you how much a nutrient in a serving of food contributes to a daily diet. 2,000 calories a day is used for general nutrition advice.

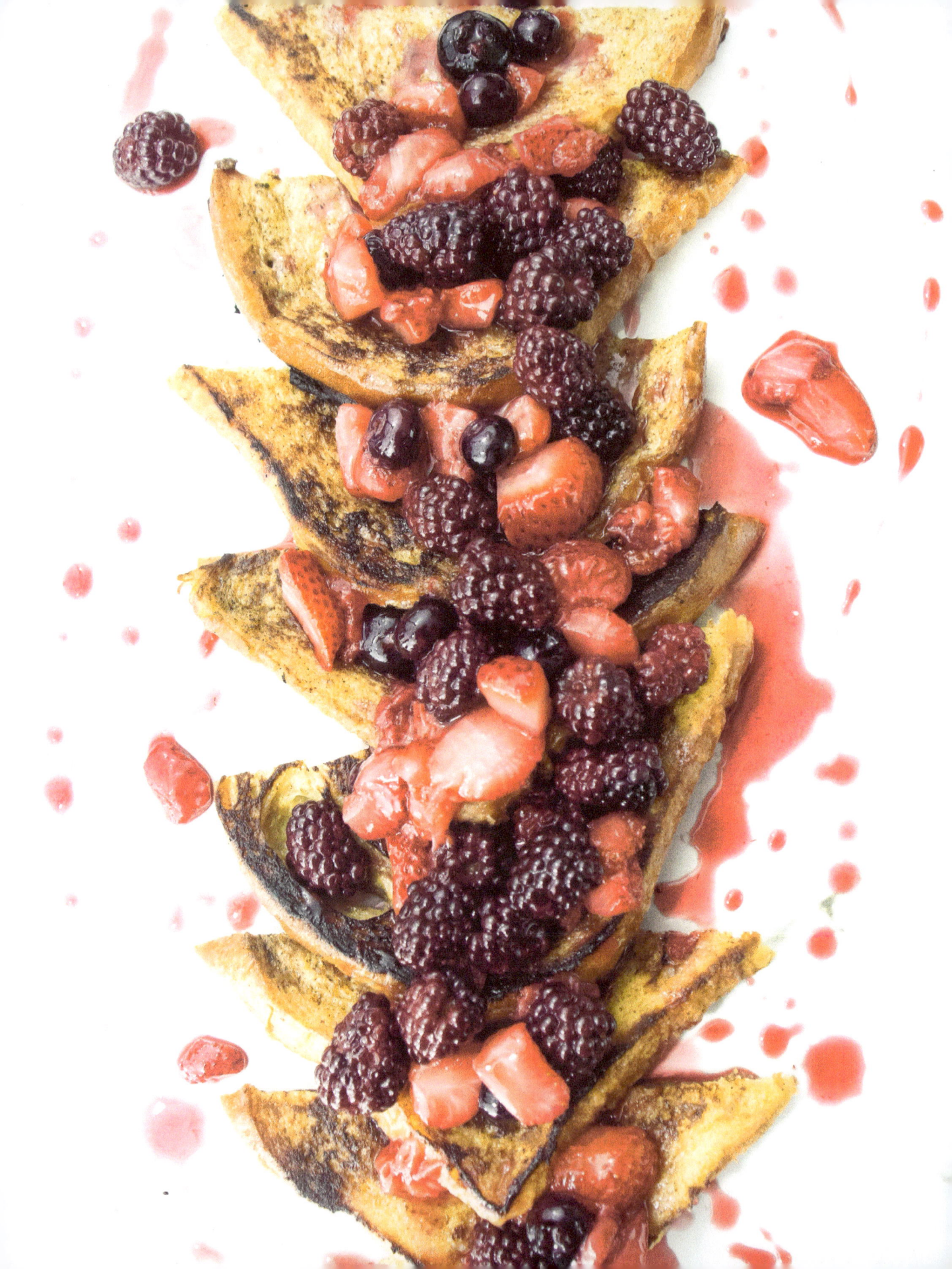

# THE "UNFORGETTABLE" FRENCH TOAST

## Ingredients:

- 2 slices of white or wheat bread
- 1 large egg
- ¼ cup vanilla almond milk
- 1 ounce French Vanilla Cîroc
- 1 teaspoon cinnamon
- 1 teaspoon of vanilla extract
- ¼ cup fresh or thawed strawberries
- ¼ cup fresh or thawed blueberries
- 3 tablespoon Sugar free syrup
- 2 tablespoon whipped cream
- Optional: Coconut flakes for garnish

Everyone deserves a treat and what's better than having a delicious serving of French Toast with friends perhaps during brunch! Whip up this French Toast, throw on some French Montana and toast with your friends for an unforgettable experience! Make Mimosas with 2 parts champagne, half ounce of vanilla Cîroc and a splash of orange juice! "Haan!" Don't forget to top your French Toast with some fruit or add berries to your Mimosa like Sammy Sousa!

## Directions:

1. Beat egg, vanilla Cîroc, and cinnamon in a shallow dish. Stir in almond milk.

2. Dip bread in egg mixture, let soak for 1 minute, turning to coat both sides evenly.

3. Cook bread slices on lightly greased nonstick griddle or skillet on medium heat until browned on both sides.

4. Garnish with ½ cup of strawberries or blueberries or blackberries with shredded coconut and serve with maple-flavored syrup.

# Nutrition Facts

1 servings per container

| Serving size | 2 Slices of French Toast |
|---|---|

| Amount Per Serving | |
|---|---|
| **Calories** | **280** |

| | % Daily Value* |
|---|---|
| **Total Fat** 8g | **10%** |
| Saturated Fat 2g | 10% |
| *Trans* Fat 0g | |
| **Cholesterol** 180mg | **60%** |
| **Sodium** 340mg | **15%** |
| **Total Carbohydrate** 36g | **13%** |
| Dietary Fiber 7g | 25% |
| Total Sugars 0g | |
| Includes 0g Added Sugars | 0% |
| **Protein** 13g | **26%** |

Not a significant source of vitamin D, calcium, iron, and potassium

* The % Daily Value (DV) tells you how much a nutrient in a serving of food contributes to a daily diet. 2,000 calories a day is used for general nutrition advice.

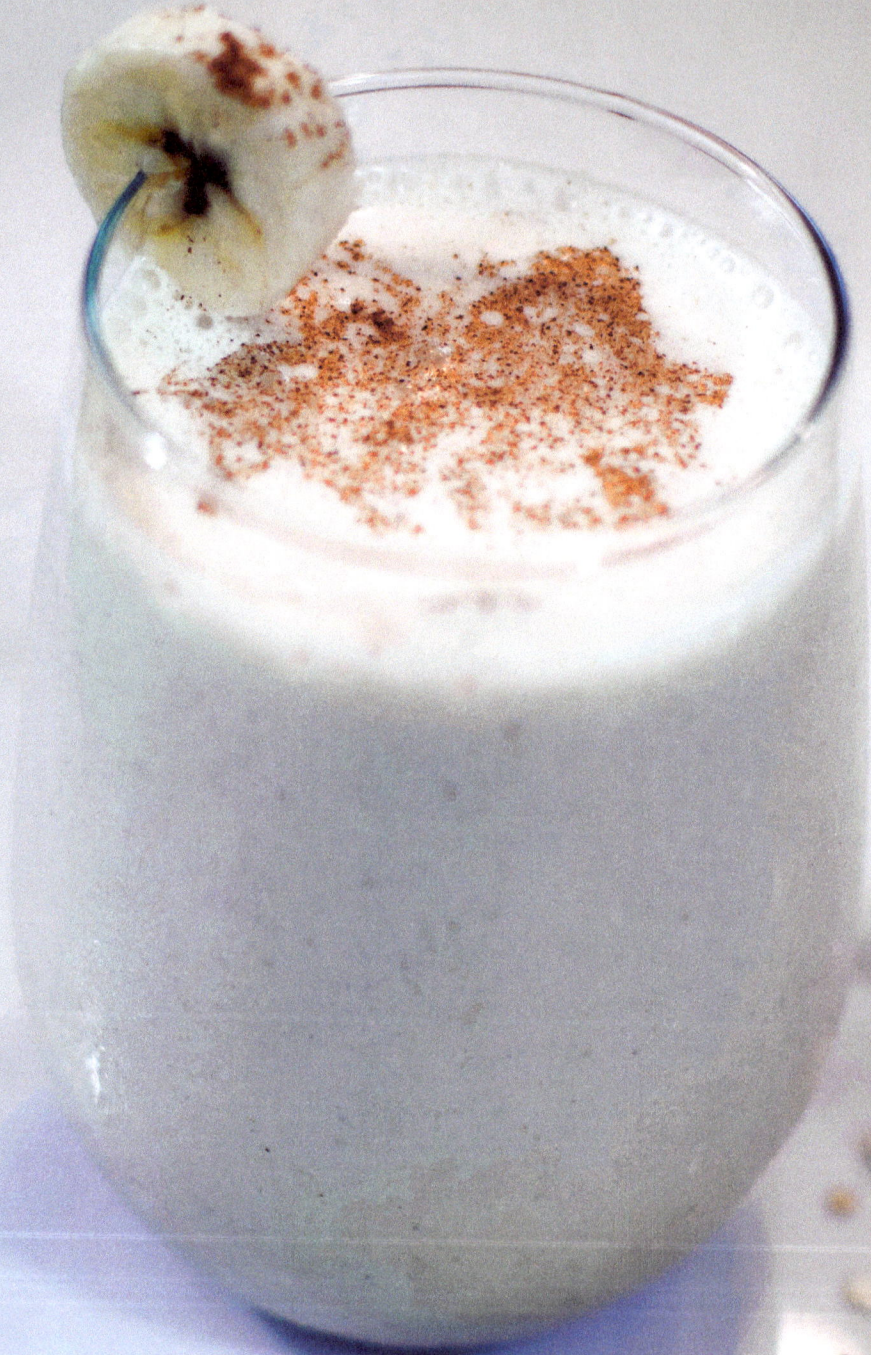

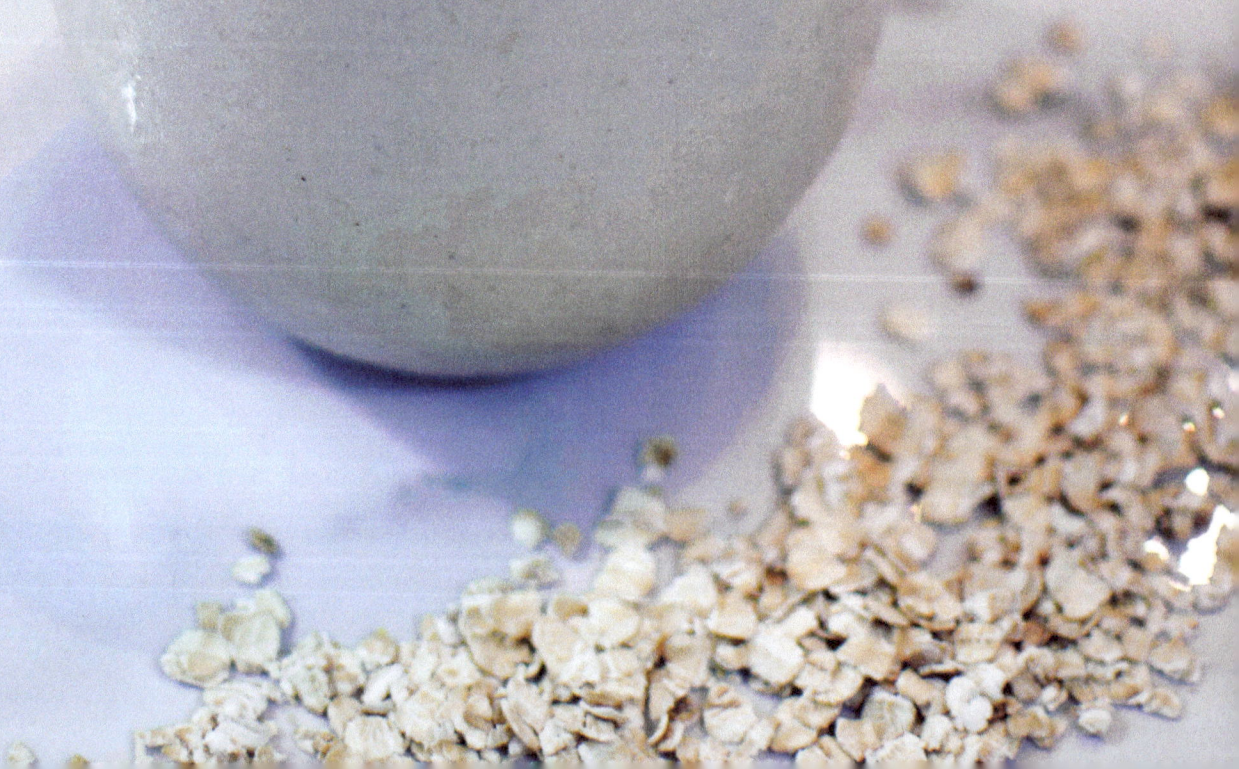

# THE "WOO-HAH!" PEANUT BUTTER BUSTA PROTEIN SHAKE

## Ingredients:

- 1 tablespoon of Natural Peanut Butter
- 8 ounce almond milk
- ¼ cup of Quick Oats, Dry
- 1 scoop of vanilla or chocolate whey protein
- ½ teaspoon cinnamon

Optional:
- 3 ice cubes or 1 teaspoon instant coffee powder or
- ¼ cup oatmeal or ½ banana

This may sound crazy, but you can mix peanut butter, whey protein, milk, cinnamon, oatmeal, and banana into the blender with some ice for a protein shake that will make you say, "woo hah!" "Give me some more!" You can modify this recipe to your liking with the foundation of the recipe being peanut butter, milk, and protein. You can choose whey protein or an alternative of your choice. Enjoy!

## Directions:

1. Use a blender to mix all ingredients

2. Add the almond, protein, peanut butter, cinnamon, and optional ingredients of your choice

3. Add ice for a thicker colder smoothie and blend for 60 seconds or until smooth and enjoy!

# Nutrition Facts

1 servings per container

| Serving size | 1 8 oz. |
|---|---|

**Amount Per Serving**

| Calories | 300 |
|---|---|

| | % Daily Value* |
|---|---|
| **Total Fat** 13g | 17% |
| Saturated Fat 2g | 10% |
| *Trans* Fat 0g | |
| **Cholesterol** 65mg | 22% |
| **Sodium** 300mg | 13% |
| **Total Carbohydrate** 17g | 6% |
| Dietary Fiber 5g | 18% |
| Total Sugars 0g | |
| Includes 0g Added Sugars | 0% |
| **Protein** 30g | 60% |

Not a significant source of vitamin D, calcium, iron, and potassium

*The % Daily Value (DV) tells you how much a nutrient in a serving of food contributes to a daily diet. 2,000 calories a day is used for general nutrition advice.

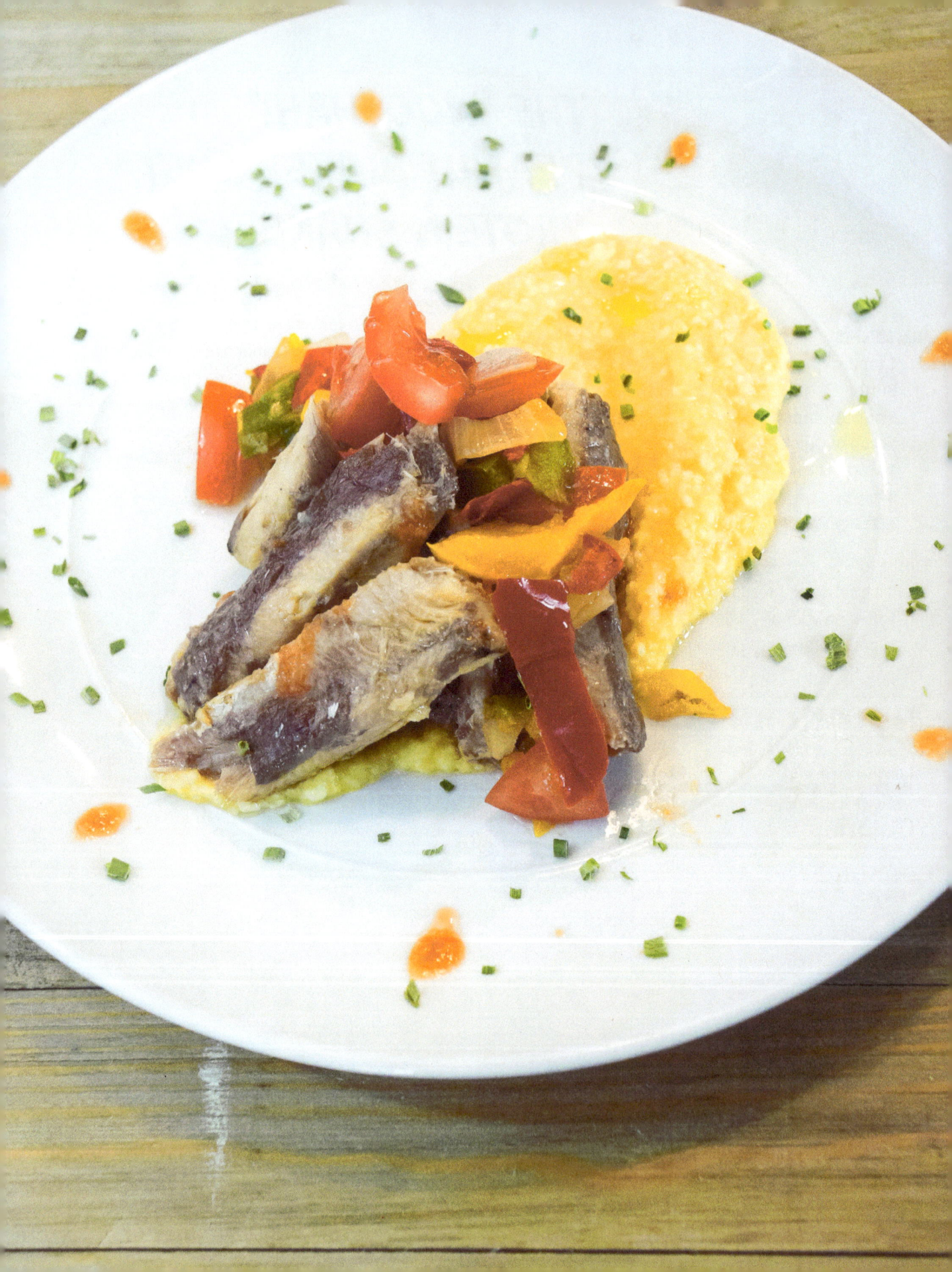

# YOU WILIN' FISH & GRITS

## Ingredients:

- 1 packet of instant grits, butter flavor, dry
- 1 can of skinless boneless sardines
- ½ cup chopped peppers, all colors
- ¼ cup chopped onion
- 1 whole egg
- Optional: 1 ounce of cheese

Sardines and grits, not for the faint of heart, but great for the heart! Sardines and grits is certainly not a popular dish; however, it is very healthy. Sardines provide protein and omega-3 fatty acids, a type of fat that reduces inflammation, lowers triglycerides, and helps to reduce the risk for heart disease. The mixture of sardines with grits makes for a surprisingly delicious dish! Add vegetables for a complete meal. Bet you never seen a dish like this!

## Directions (makes one serving):

1. Heat skillet with non-stick spray
2. Add fresh or frozen vegetables to pan and sauté
3. Add egg and scramble
4. Add one packet of grits to a bowl with a ½ c of water, heat in microwave for 2 minutes
5. Add vegetables and eggs to grits, open can of sardines, drain oil and add to bowl, mix, and garnish with tomatoes!

## Nutrition Facts

1 servings per container

| Serving size | 1 bowl |
|---|---|

**Amount Per Serving**

| Calories | 490 |
|---|---|

| | % Daily Value* |
|---|---|
| **Total Fat** 25g | **32%** |
| Saturated Fat 8g | **40%** |
| *Trans* Fat 0g | |
| **Cholesterol** 260mg | **87%** |
| **Sodium** 1010mg | **44%** |
| **Total Carbohydrate** 32g | **12%** |
| Dietary Fiber 3g | **11%** |
| Total Sugars 0g | |
| Includes 0g Added Sugars | **0%** |
| **Protein** 37g | **74%** |

Not a significant source of vitamin D, calcium, iron, and potassium

* The % Daily Value (DV) tells you how much a nutrient in a serving of food contributes to a daily diet. 2,000 calories a day is used for general nutrition advice.

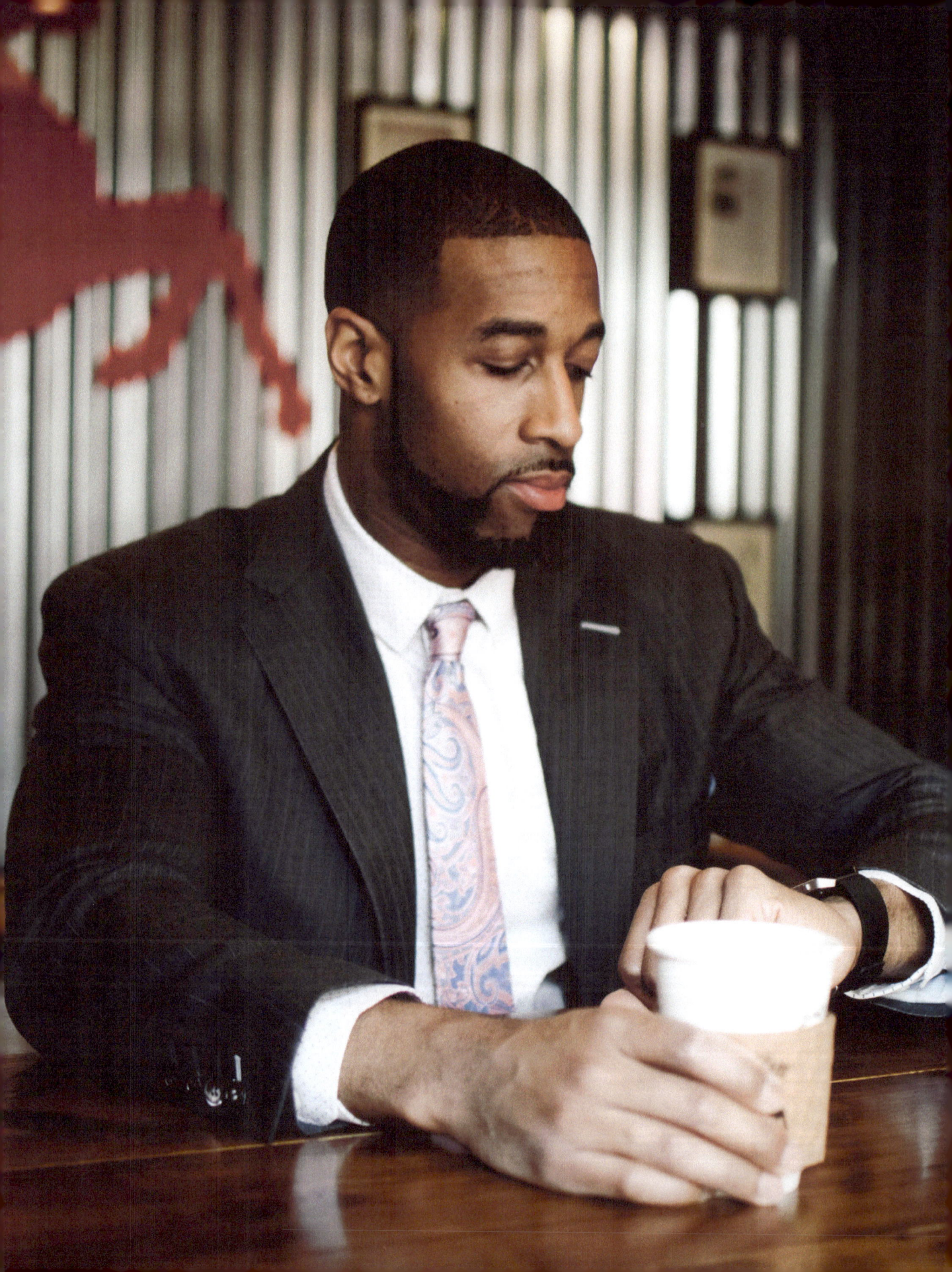

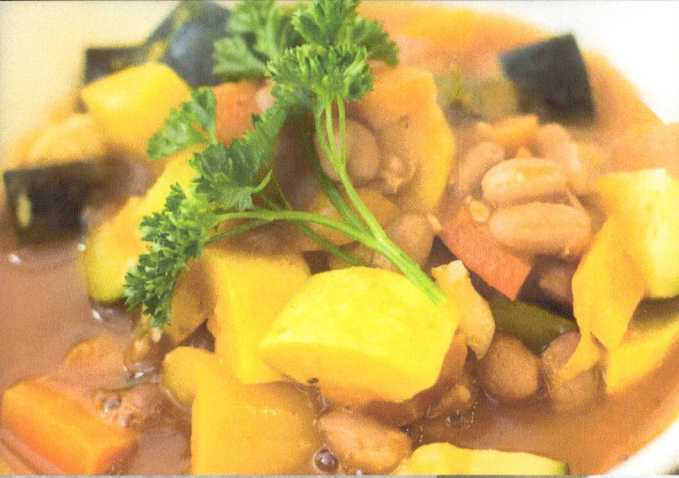

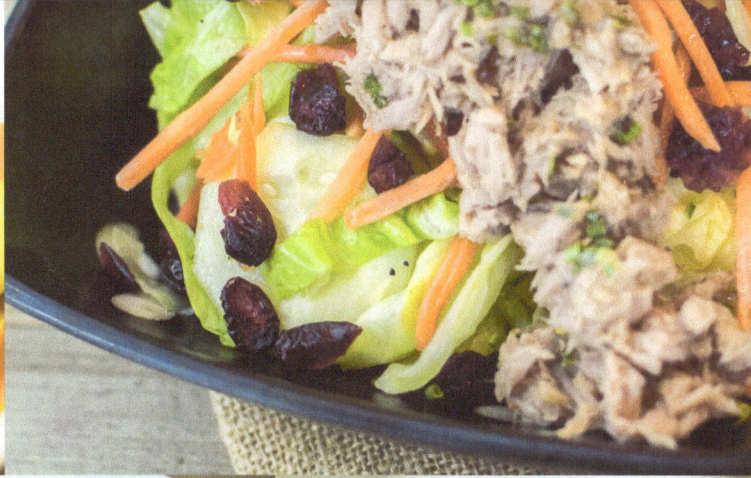

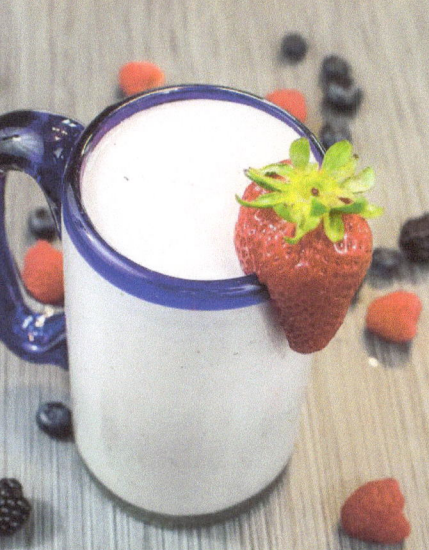

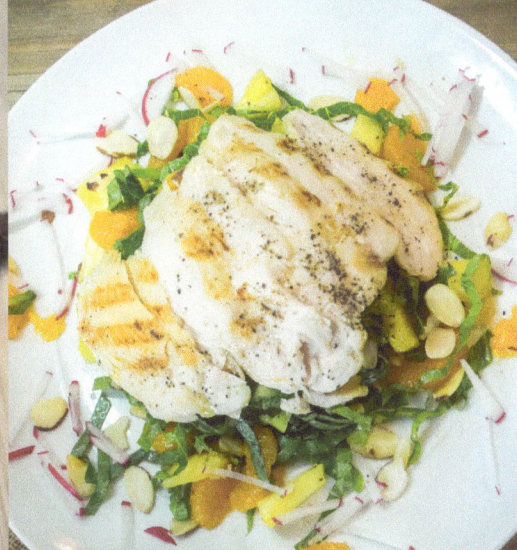

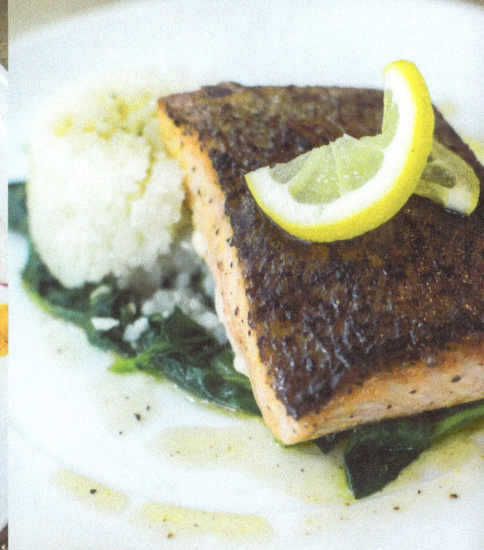

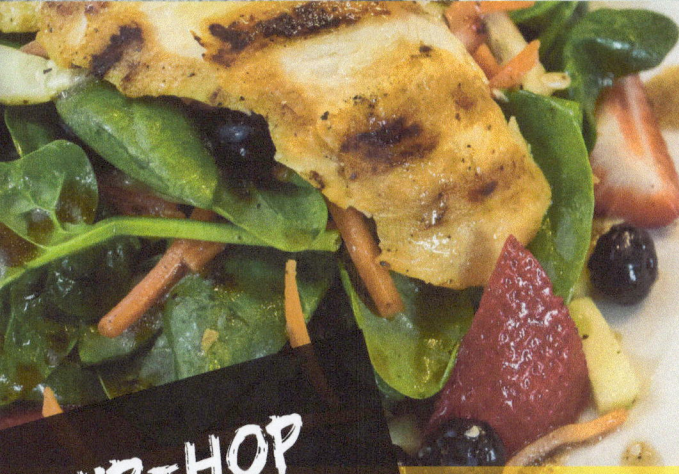

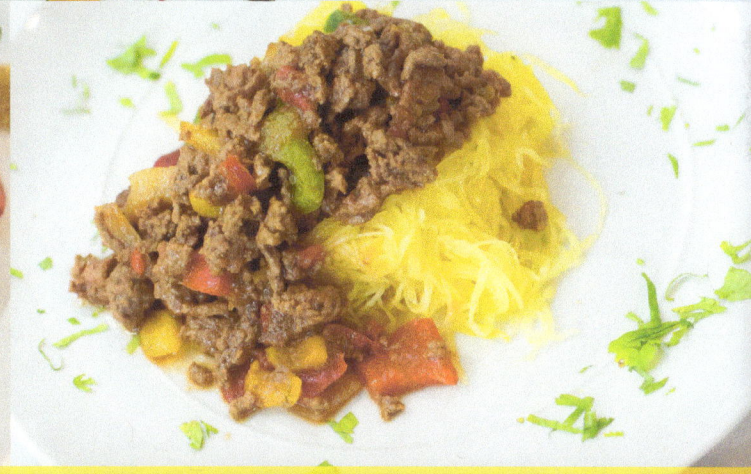

Lunch can either make or break the day! Knowing what you will have beforehand, packing your lunch or eating a good breakfast to sustain your appetite is important so that you are mindful of the food choices you will make which can help with calorie control. Here are some healthy hip-hop nspired lunch options for you to choose.

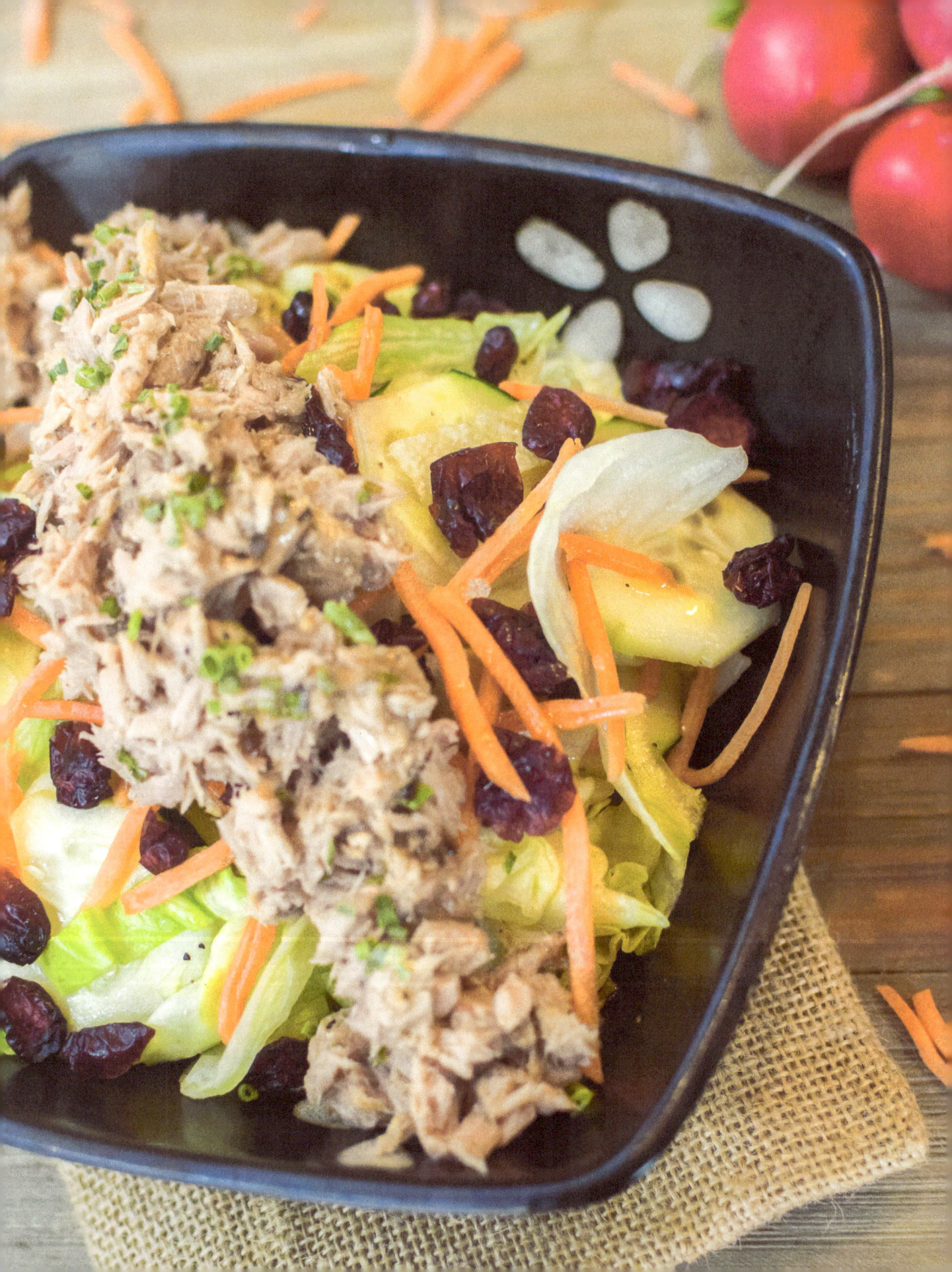

## TRACK 8

# TOO GOOD TUNA SALAD

## Ingredients:

- 2 cups of spring lettuce
- 1 can light chunk tuna
- 2 tablespoons of light balsamic dressing
- ¼ cup shredded carrots
- ½ cup cucumbers
- ¼ cup chopped tomatoes
- 1 ounce dried Craisins

This tuna salad is too good and healthy too. This salad is rich in leafy greens, high in fiber and lycopene, an antioxidant found in tomatoes to help reduce the risk of prostate cancer. The tuna is also a great source of protein and omega 3 fatty acids. Toss and add the dressing of choice. I would recommend using light vinaigrette based dressing's verses creamy dressing to reduce calories. You can also consider adding more fruit such as strawberries or mango for a tropical delicious tasting twist!

## Directions (makes one salad):

1. Add all ingredients in a mixing bowl, toss add dressing and serve

## Nutrition Facts

1 servings per container

| Serving size | 1 salad |
|---|---|

**Amount Per Serving**

| **Calories** | **290** |
|---|---|

| | % Daily Value* |
|---|---|
| **Total Fat** 6g | **8%** |
| Saturated Fat 1g | **5%** |
| *Trans* Fat 0g | |
| **Cholesterol** 50mg | **17%** |
| **Sodium** 600mg | **26%** |
| **Total Carbohydrate** 14g | **5%** |
| Dietary Fiber 4g | **14%** |
| Total Sugars 0g | |
| Includes 0g Added Sugars | **0%** |
| **Protein** 44g | **88%** |

Not a significant source of vitamin D, calcium, iron, and potassium

* The % Daily Value (DV) tells you how much a nutrient in a serving of food contributes to a daily diet. 2,000 calories a day is used for general nutrition advice.

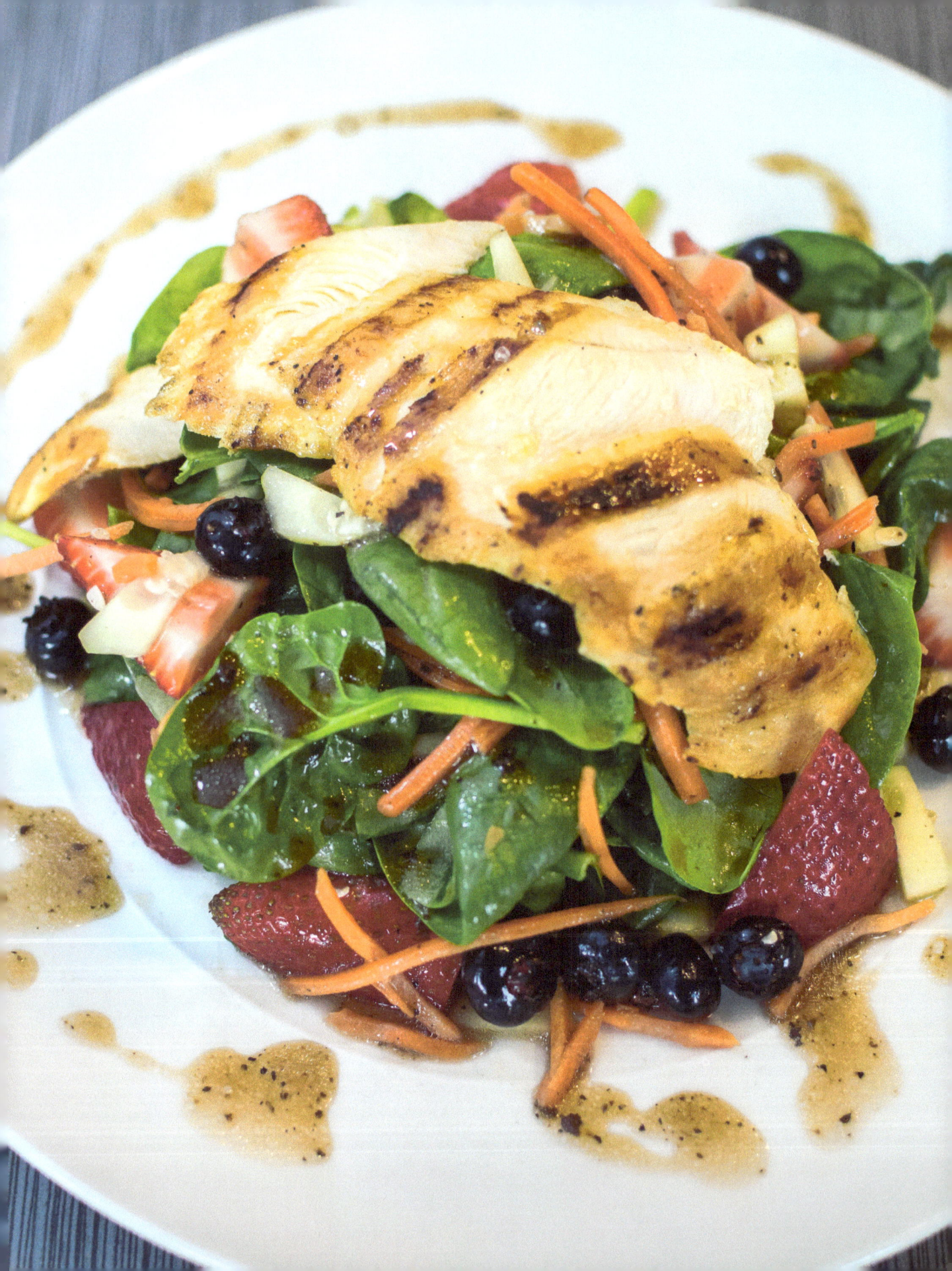

*Inspired by:*
**DRAKE,
"FANCY"**

# "FANCY" SPINACH CHICKEN SALAD

## Ingredients:

- 2 cups spinach
- 6 ounces grilled chicken
- ¼ cup shredded carrots
- ½ cup sliced cucumbers
- ¼ cup cherry tomatoes
- ½ cup strawberries and blueberries
- Optional: 1 ounce walnuts

This "fancy" spinach chicken salad calls for spinach as the base of the meal. The darker leafy green will provide more nutrients than the typical Iceberg lettuce. The grilled chicken will provide an excellent source of protein, but if you're vegetarian you can substitute with tofu or beans or nuts and seeds. Stay fancy and healthy with this simple, delicious, nutritious hip hop dish!

## Directions (makes one salad):

1. Spray non-stick pan with olive oil and heat skillet on medium high

2. Season chicken and grill each side for about 6-7 minutes

3. Add all ingredients in a mixing bowl, toss and add dressing

## Nutrition Facts

1 servings per container

| Serving size | 1 salad |
|---|---|

**Amount Per Serving**

**Calories** **410**

| | % Daily Value* |
|---|---|
| **Total Fat** 13g | **17%** |
| Saturated Fat 3g | **15%** |
| *Trans* Fat 0g | |
| **Cholesterol** 265mg | **88%** |
| **Sodium** 920mg | **40%** |
| **Total Carbohydrate** 29g | **11%** |
| Dietary Fiber 11g | **39%** |
| Total Sugars 0g | |
| Includes 0g Added Sugars | **0%** |
| **Protein** 50g | **100%** |

Not a significant source of vitamin D, calcium, iron, and potassium

*The % Daily Value (DV) tells you how much a nutrient in a serving of food contributes to a daily diet. 2,000 calories a day is used for general nutrition advice.

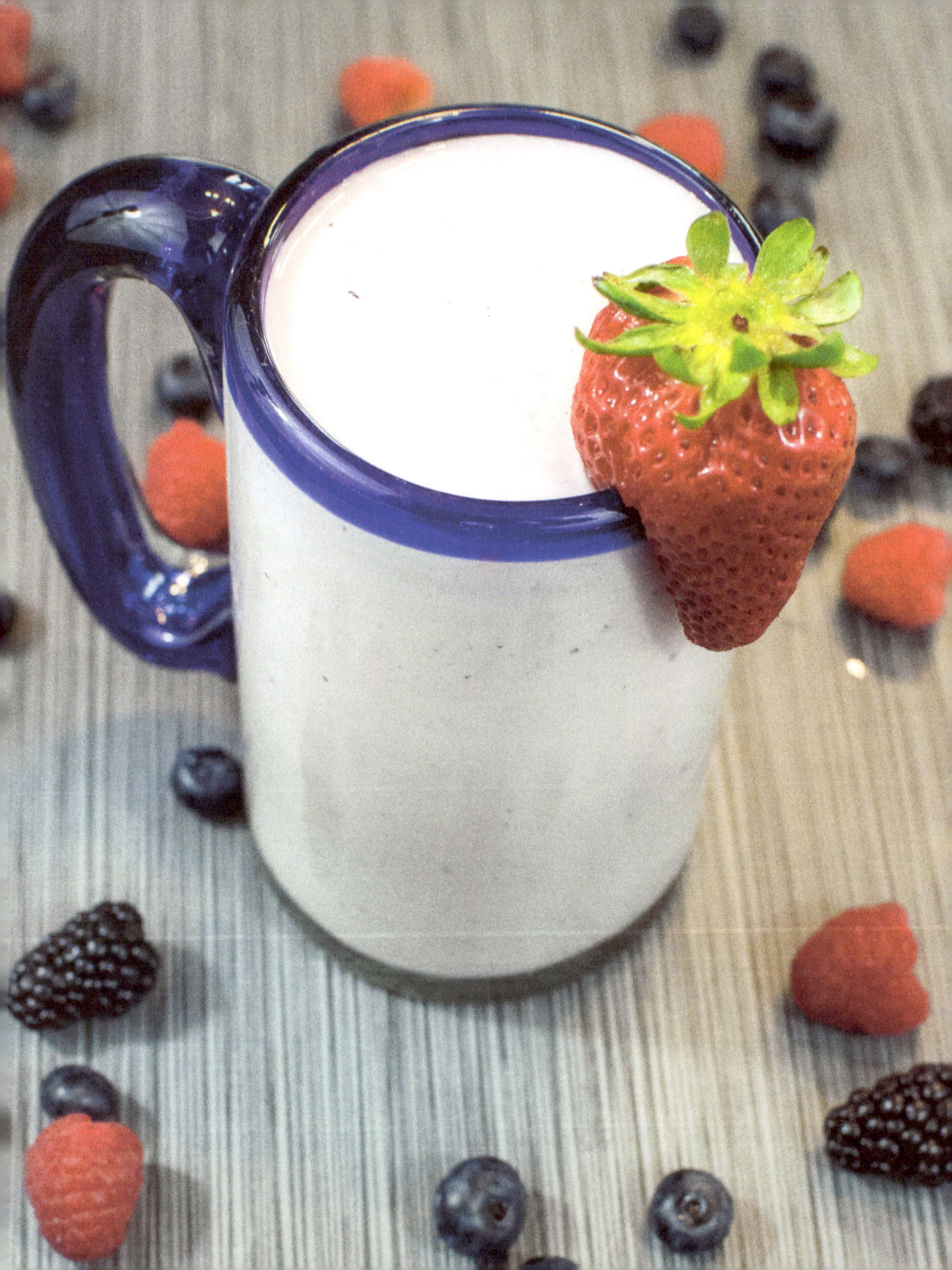

# SUPER BASS BERRY MINAJ SHAKE

## Ingredients:

- 4 ounces almond milk or water or fat-free milk
- 8 ounces Vanilla Greek yogurt
- 1 cup fresh or frozen blackberries, blueberries & strawberries
- 1 scoop of whey protein
- Garnish with mint

Protein shakes can fit at any time of the day. Try this Super Bass Berry Minaj Shake as a quick lunch option. This shake is rich in powerful like tones of antioxidants to give it that super berry bass blast! It provides the perfect minaj of Greek yogurt and berries for a simple, delicious, nutritious smoothie. The whey protein can be optional and helps to increase the protein content to keep you fuller, and support muscle and weight loss. You may choose the protein supplement of your choice.

## Directions (makes one protein shake):

1. Use your blender to mix all ingredients

2. Add the almond milk, yogurt, berries, and whey protein

3. Add ice for a thicker colder smoothie and blend for 60 seconds or until smooth and enjoy!

## Nutrition Facts

1 servings per container

| Serving size | 16 oz |
|---|---|

**Amount Per Serving**

| Calories | 330 |
|---|---|

| | % Daily Value* |
|---|---|
| **Total Fat** 4g | 5% |
| Saturated Fat 1g | 5% |
| *Trans* Fat 0g | |
| **Cholesterol** 75mg | 25% |
| **Sodium** 220mg | 10% |
| **Total Carbohydrate** 31g | 11% |
| Dietary Fiber 6g | 21% |
| Total Sugars 0g | |
| Includes 0g Added Sugars | 0% |
| **Protein** 42g | 84% |

Not a significant source of vitamin D, calcium, iron, and potassium

*The % Daily Value (DV) tells you how much a nutrient in a serving of food contributes to a daily diet. 2,000 calories a day is used for general nutrition advice.

# WILD SALMON, SPINACH, AND CAULIFLOWER

## Ingredients:

- 6 ounces wild salmon
- 4 cups fresh spinach
- 1 teaspoon garlic salt
- 1 teaspoon lemon pepper seasoning
- 1 tablespoon garlic
- 2 tablespoons extra virgin olive oil
- 1 cup of mashed cauliflower (commercially available microwavable)
- 1 teaspoon dill
- 1 lemon wedge

This is a wildly nutritious meal for you to eat at least twice per week. The American Heart Association recommends two fish meals per week. Salmon is another excellent source of omega 3 fatty acids that is good for heart health, and brain health (supports memory). The mashed cauliflower is an excellent alternative to mashed potatoes (although the choice is yours!). Make it a wild and memorable experience!

## Directions (makes one serving):

1. Heat medium sized pan with 1 tablespoon of olive oil

2. Add spinach while pan is heating up, toss and season with garlic salt and cover, cook and toss occasionally for 8 minutes.

3. In a separate medium sized non-stick pan heat 1 tablespoon of olive oil with garlic

4. Season salmon with lemon pepper seasoning and grill both sides for approximately 5 minutes each

5. Microwave Birds Eye Steamfresh Veggie Made™ Mashed Cauliflower Original for 5 minutes

6. Plate ingredients and enjoy!

# Nutrition Facts

1 servings per container

| | |
|---|---|
| **Serving size** | **1 Wild Salmon, Spinach** |

**Amount Per Serving**

| **Calories** | **630** |
|---|---|

| | % Daily Value* |
|---|---|
| **Total Fat** 45g | **58%** |
| Saturated Fat 10g | **50%** |
| *Trans* Fat 0g | |
| **Cholesterol** 115mg | **38%** |
| **Sodium** 2260mg | **98%** |
| **Total Carbohydrate** 20g | **7%** |
| Dietary Fiber 9g | **32%** |
| Total Sugars 0g | |
| Includes 0g Added Sugars | **0%** |
| **Protein** 42g | **84%** |

Not a significant source of vitamin D, calcium, iron, and potassium

*The % Daily Value (DV) tells you how much a nutrient in a serving of food contributes to a daily diet. 2,000 calories a day is used for general nutrition advice.

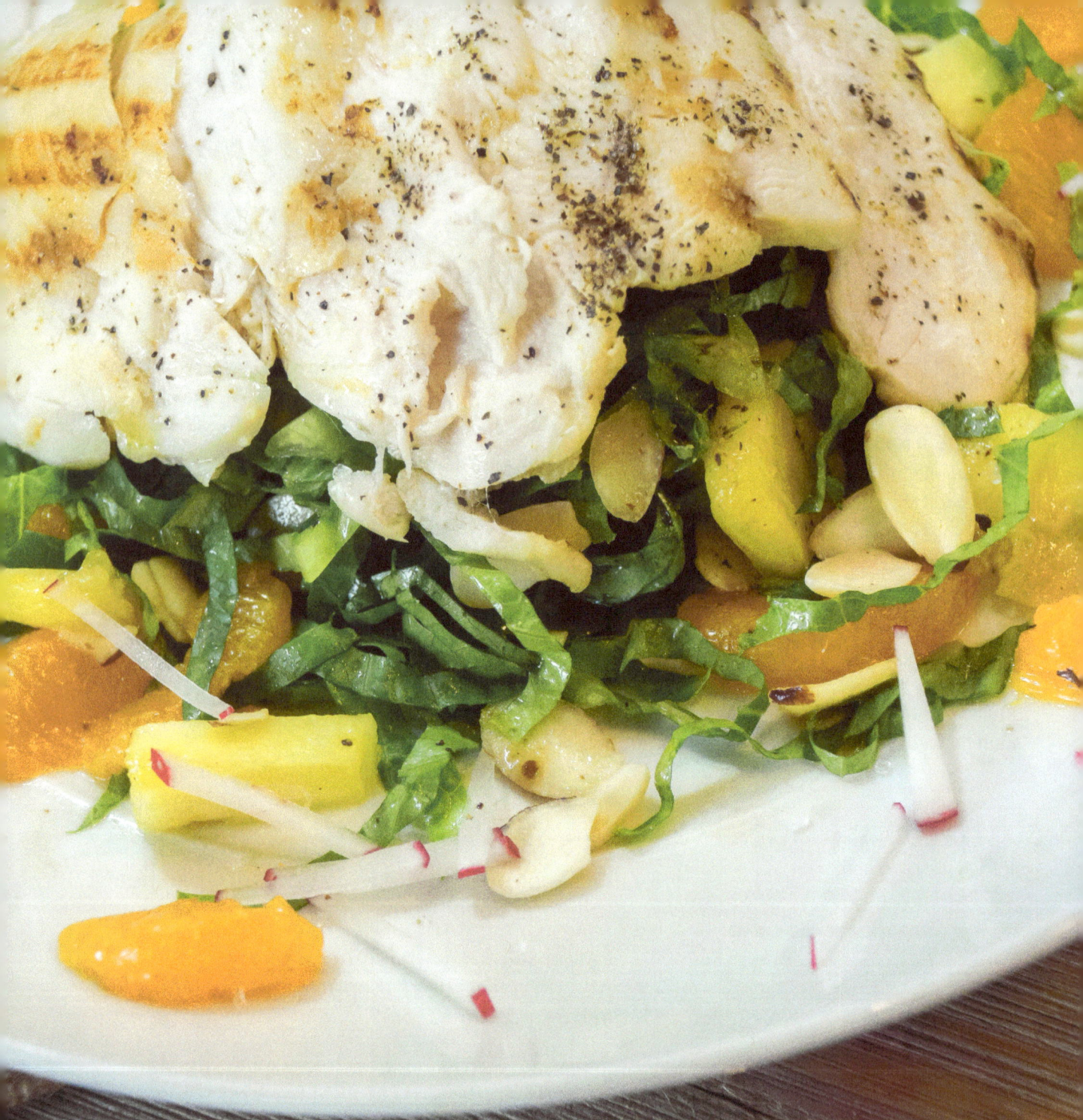

# RICK'S "DICED PINEAPPLE" CHICKEN SALAD

## Ingredients:

- 1 lb. boneless, skinless chicken breasts
- ¼ to ½ cup slivered almonds
- 1 can mandarin oranges, drained
- 1 can diced pineapple chunks, drained and rinsed
- Head of lettuce

Pineapples contain an enzyme known as bromelain which can help to reduce heart burn and act as a nasal decongestant. Pineapples are also an excellent source of vitamin C to help support immunity. Choose fresh or frozen and thaw depending on the time of year. If you choose canned be sure to rinse before consumption to reduce the amount of sugar. I'm sure you will admire the taste!

## Directions (makes four servings):

1. Boil to simmer chicken in 1 cup of water in a covered pan for about 20 minutes, or until juices run clear when pricked with a fork.

2. Cool chicken, then dice and place in a large bowl.

3. Add pineapples, mandarin oranges and almonds to the bowl and mix.

4. Toss with dressing of choice.

5. Add ingredients over a bed of lettuce and enjoy!

## Nutrition Facts

1 servings per container

| | |
|---|---|
| **Serving size** | **1 Salad** |

**Amount Per Serving**

**Calories** **210**

| | % Daily Value* |
|---|---|
| **Total Fat** 7g | **9%** |
| Saturated Fat 1g | **5%** |
| *Trans* Fat 0g | |
| **Cholesterol** 65mg | **22%** |
| **Sodium** 1560mg | **68%** |
| **Total Carbohydrate** 9g | **3%** |
| Dietary Fiber 2g | **7%** |
| Total Sugars 0g | |
| Includes 0g Added Sugars | **0%** |
| **Protein** 28g | **56%** |

Not a significant source of vitamin D, calcium, iron, and potassium

* The % Daily Value (DV) tells you how much a nutrient in a serving of food contributes to a daily diet. 2,000 calories a day is used for general nutrition advice.

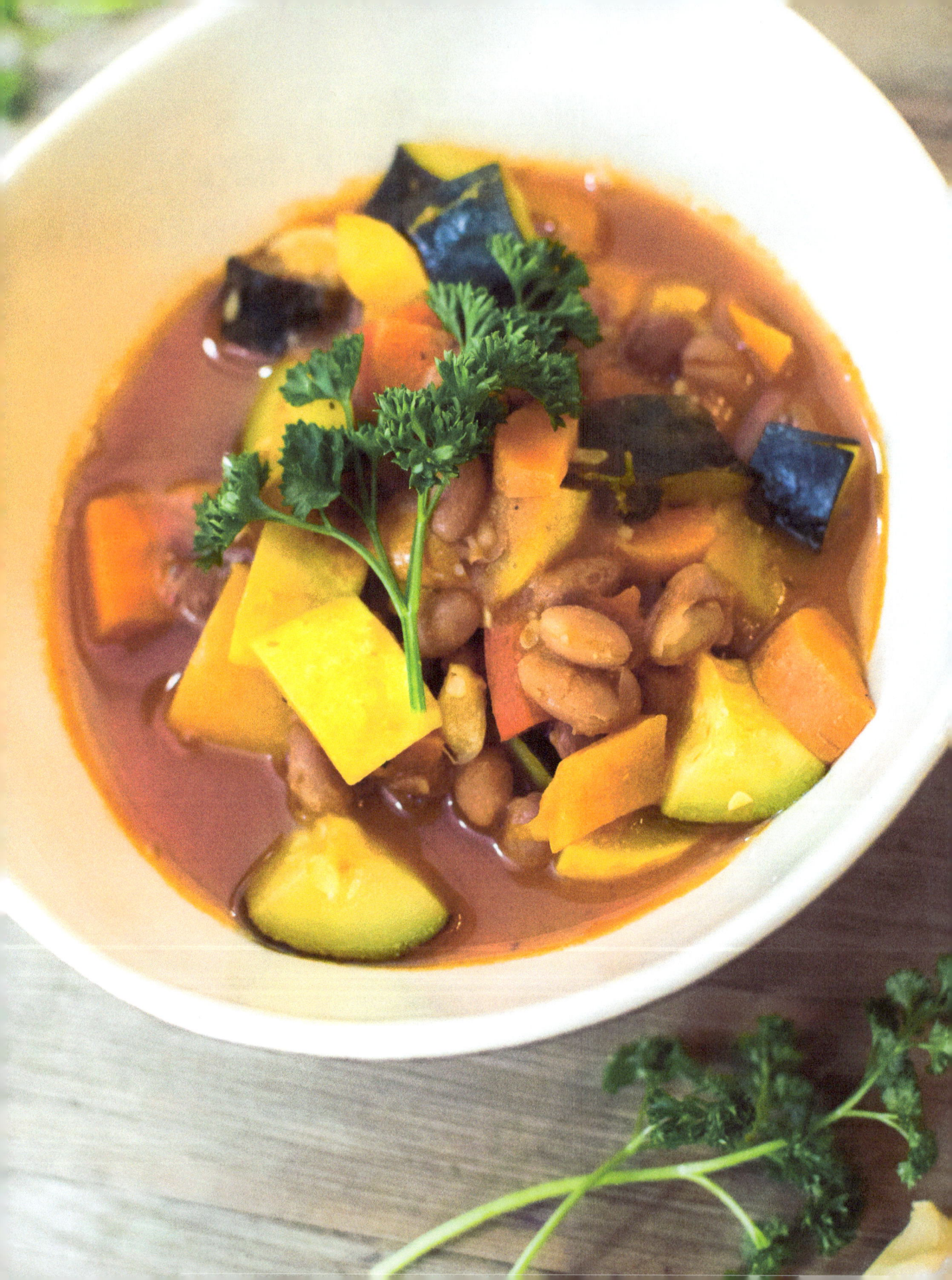

# "NEEDED ME" VEGETABLE MEDLEY

## Ingredients:

- 1 cup sliced zucchini squash
- 1 cup carrot sticks
- 1 cup of frozen ready tri color pepper & onion blend
- ½ cup pink beans
- 1 tablespoon chopped garlic
- ½ cup canned tomato sauce
- 2 teaspoons parsley
- 1 teaspoon salt
- ½ cup water

According to the Centers for Disease Control (CDC) in 2015 only 1 in 10 Americans eats enough fruits and vegetables. We need fruits and vegetables to fight disease. If you are not consuming the recommended 5 servings per day (which is modest) then your risk and probability of developing chronic diseases such as obesity, heart disease and diabetes increase. Fruits and vegetables are low in calories, high in fiber and rich in phytonutrients to help fight disease. You need your fruits and vegetables. Vegetable medley will meet 3 out of 5 of your daily vegetable needs!

## Directions:

1. Heat butter and garlic over medium heat

2. Add all vegetables, corn and season with salt and pepper, sauté and stir

3. Add tomato sauce with ½ cup water with parsley

4. Simmer for 8 minutes and serve!

## Nutrition Facts

1 servings per container

| Serving size | 8 oz |
|---|---|

**Amount Per Serving**

| Calories | 340 |
|---|---|

| | % Daily Value* |
|---|---|
| **Total Fat** 11g | **14%** |
| Saturated Fat 2g | **10%** |
| *Trans* Fat 0g | |
| **Cholesterol** 0mg | **0%** |
| **Sodium** 2740mg | **119%** |
| **Total Carbohydrate** 52g | **19%** |
| Dietary Fiber 12g | **43%** |
| Total Sugars 0g | |
| Includes 0g Added Sugars | **0%** |
| **Protein** 12g | **24%** |

Not a significant source of vitamin D, calcium, iron, and potassium

* The % Daily Value (DV) tells you how much a nutrient in a serving of food contributes to a daily diet. 2,000 calories a day is used for general nutrition advice.

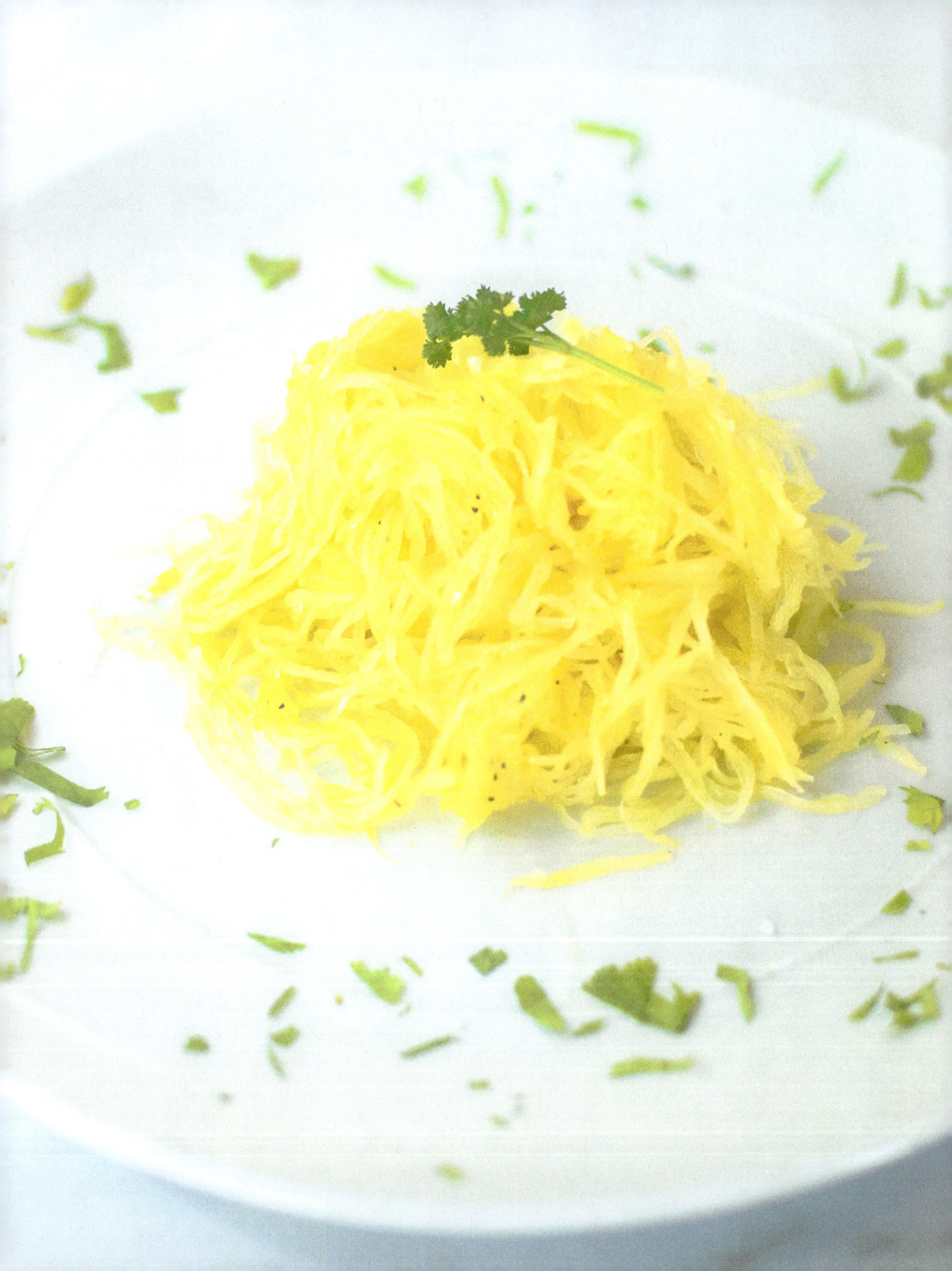

# SPAGHETTI SQUASH & JOE

## Ingredients:

- 1 cup spaghetti squash
- 1 tablespoon chopped garlic
- ½ teaspoon salt
- ½ teaspoon pepper
- 1 tablespoon olive oil
- 1 cup of leftover "Damn" turkey Chili

Spaghetti, pasta, noodles, ziti it's all carbohydrates in different shapes and sizes. We often have a high intake of carbohydrates with our spaghetti dish! Carbohydrates are necessary to fuel muscle for athletes, but most of the population is more than plenty fueled with carbohydrate rich foods. This recipe is designed to cut down on the carbs to create more balance, moderation, support of health, wellness, and weight loss. This recipe provides about 15 g of carbohydrate per serving and will likely reduce your typical carbohydrate intake by more than half, which means less calories and more potential for a healthy waistline, weight maintenance or lean body mass gains when adding a resistance training regimen on top of a healthy, well balanced protein laden diet! Add the "Damn" turkey chili for an additional 29 grams of muscle building protein!

## Nutrition Facts

1 servings per container

**Serving size** 8 oz

**Amount Per Serving**

**Calories** 190

| | % Daily Value* |
|---|---|
| **Total Fat** 15g | 19% |
| Saturated Fat 2g | 10% |
| *Trans* Fat 0g | |
| **Cholesterol** 0mg | 0% |
| **Sodium** 1560mg | 68% |
| **Total Carbohydrate** 15g | 5% |
| Dietary Fiber 3g | 11% |
| Total Sugars 0g | |
| Includes 0g Added Sugars | 0% |
| **Protein** 2g | 4% |

Not a significant source of vitamin D, calcium, iron, and potassium

*The % Daily Value (DV) tells you how much a nutrient in a serving of food contributes to a daily diet. 2,000 calories a day is used for general nutrition advice.

## Directions:

1. Preheat oven to 350-375ºF.

2. Halve raw spaghetti squash with a sturdy sharp knife, scoop out, and discard the squash poop with a spoon.

3. Place halves onto an oven safe cooking dish face up. Add chopped garlic, salt, pepper, and olive oil.

4. Place onto the upper middle rack of the oven for about 30-40 minutes. (You will know it is ready when the squash separates with little resistance from the skin).

5. Remove from oven, and place in coldest location possible for at least 20 minutes, before separating from skin.

6. Use a fork to scoop and separate squash strands; add turkey chili and serve!

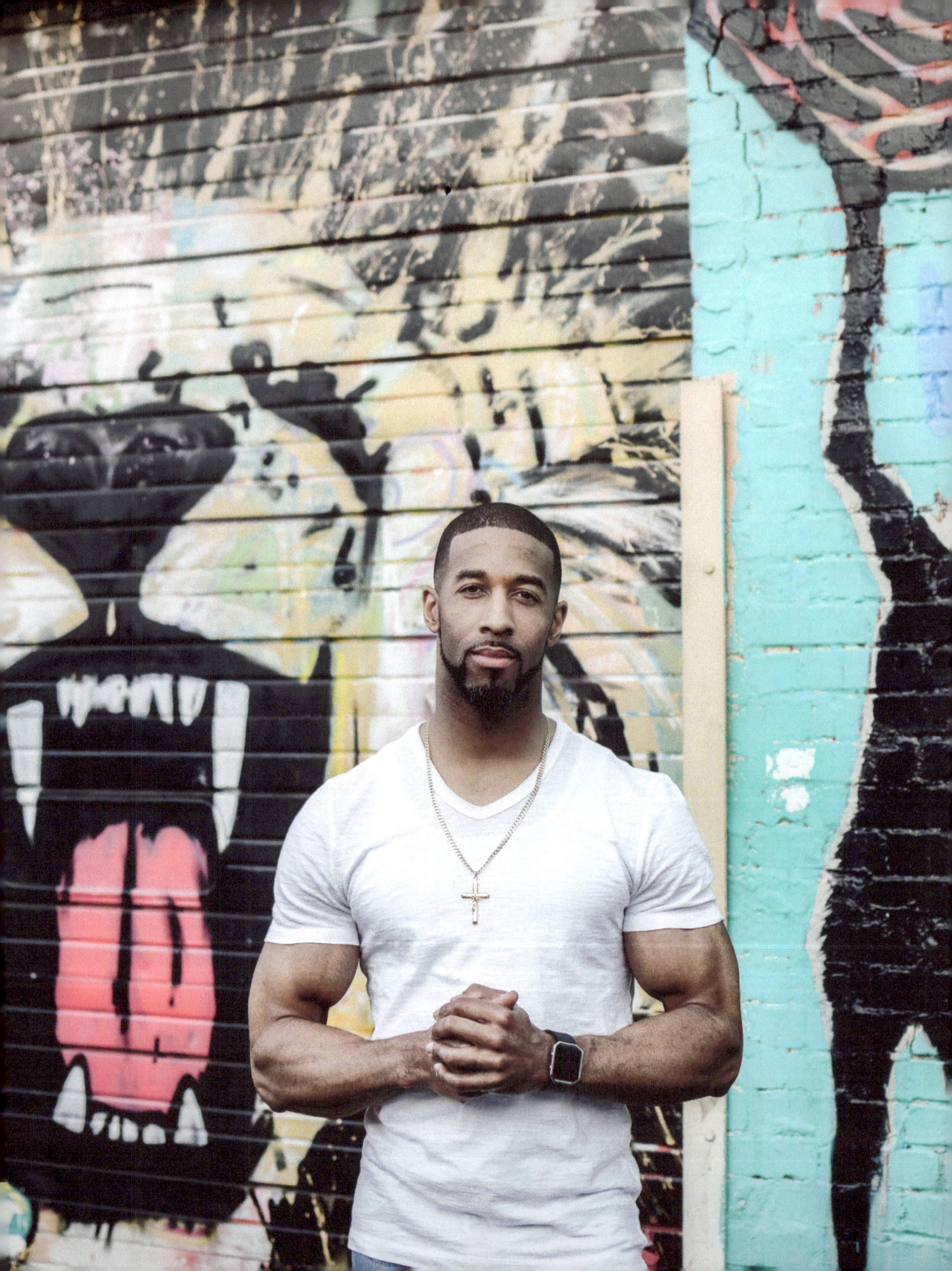

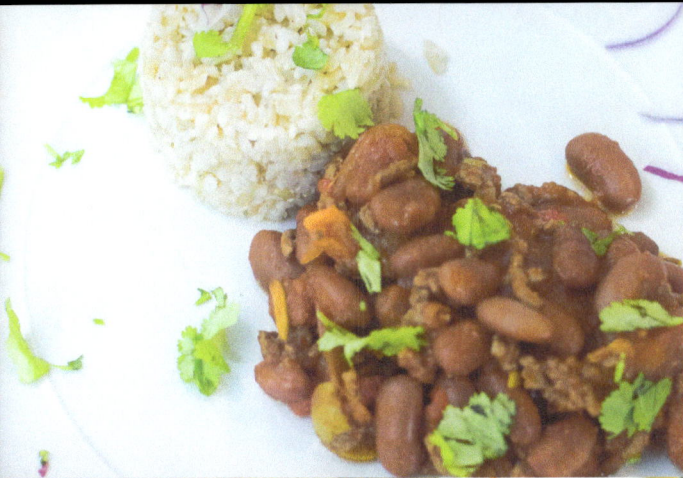

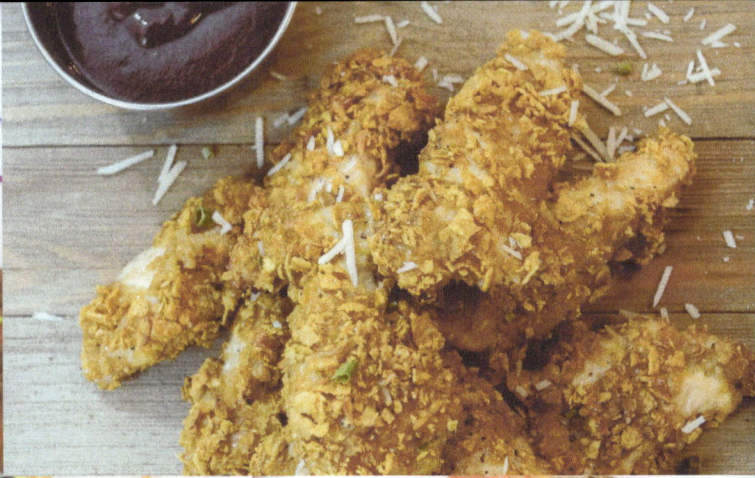

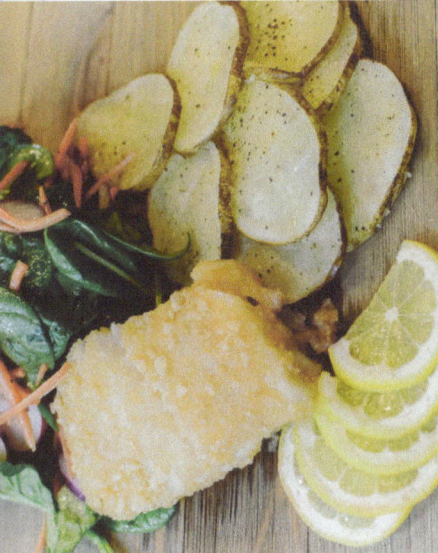

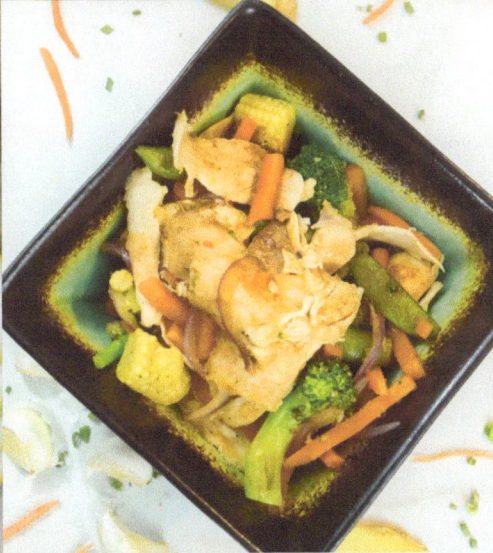

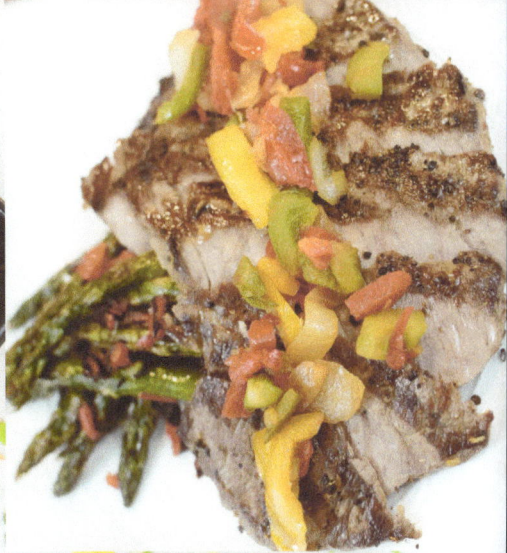

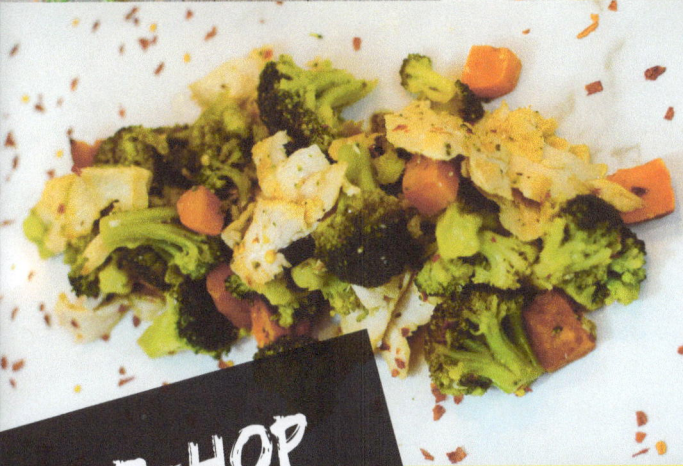

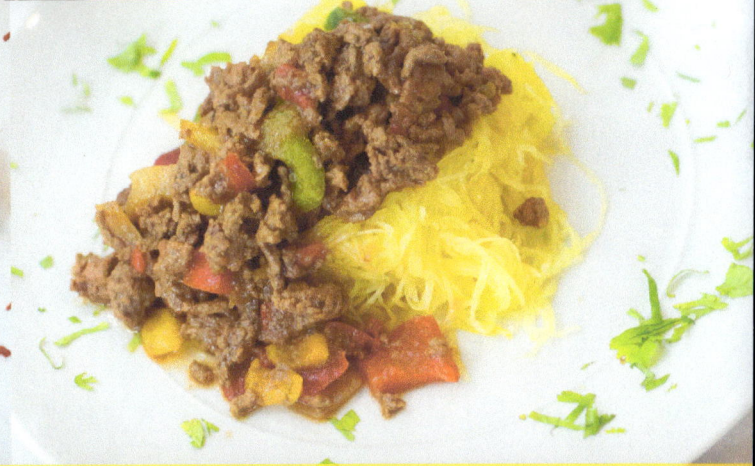

# HIP-HOP HEALTHY DINNER RECIPES

These hip-hop healthy recipes are simple, delicious, and nutritious! Feel free to make a serving or two of some of your favorite dishes without over indulging on your calorie limits. Make sure to apply the plate method (cover 50% of your plate with non-starchy vegetable, 25% with protein and 25% with carbohydrates) for a well-balanced meal.

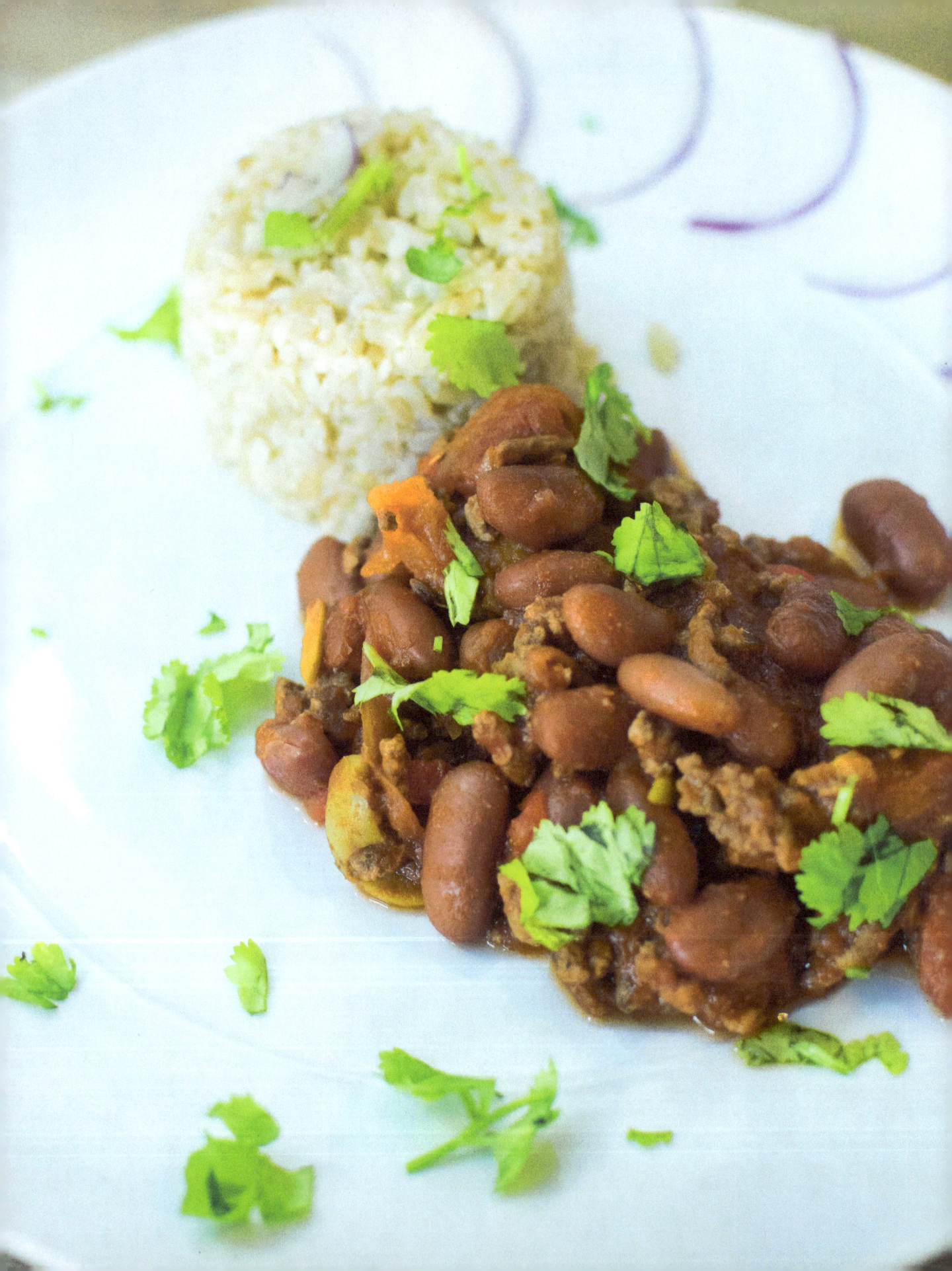

# "MI GENTE" RICE & BEANS

Me gusta arroz y habichuelas! Who doesn't love a good dish of rice and beans? This is a staple of many Latin dishes. The rice and beans make a complete protein, rich in fiber, B vitamins and potassium. Enjoy with or without added meat. Use brown or white rice, they will essentially provide the same number of calories, but the brown rice will provide more fiber and nutrients to keep you fuller. Are you with me, mi gente?

## Ingredients:

- 1 lb. of 90% lean ground beef
- 1 tablespoon. cider vinegar
- ½ cup chopped onions (fresh or frozen)
- ½ cup chopped peppers (fresh or frozen)
- ½ cup diced tomatoes
- ½ cup water
- ¼ teaspoon ground cumin
- 1 ½ teaspoon All-Purpose Seasoning with Pepper
- 1 tablespoon garlic
- 2 tablespoon extra-virgin olive oil
- 1 packet Sazon with Coriander and Annatto
- ½ cup Sofrito
- 1 bag of Whole Grain Brown Rice
- 1 can of kidney beans
- Optional: ¼ cup sliced Manzanilla Olives Stuffed with Pimientos

## Nutrition Facts

2 servings per container

| Serving size | 8 oz |
|---|---|

**Amount Per Serving**

| Calories | 420 |
|---|---|

| | % Daily Value* |
|---|---|
| **Total Fat** 22g | 28% |
| Saturated Fat 5g | 25% |
| *Trans* Fat 0g | |
| **Cholesterol** 95mg | 32% |
| **Sodium** 670mg | 29% |
| **Total Carbohydrate** 24g | 9% |
| Dietary Fiber 5g | 18% |
| Total Sugars 0g | |
| Includes 0g Added Sugars | 0% |
| **Protein** 31g | 62% |

Not a significant source of vitamin D, calcium, iron, and potassium

\* The % Daily Value (DV) tells you how much a nutrient in a serving of food contributes to a daily diet. 2,000 calories a day is used for general nutrition advice.

## Directions (makes two servings):

1. Heat oil in a 12" non-stick skillet over medium-high heat.

2. Add chopped onions, peppers, garlic to pan.

3. Season beef with ground cumin, Adobo, Sazon and add to pan. Cook until golden brown.

4. Add sofrito, tomato sauce, diced tomatoes, olives (optional) and ½ c of water

5. Open can of kidney beans, rinse and add to pan, stir, and cover on low heat for about 5-10 minutes.

6. Cook brown rice in microwave, remove and serve. Makes 4 servings

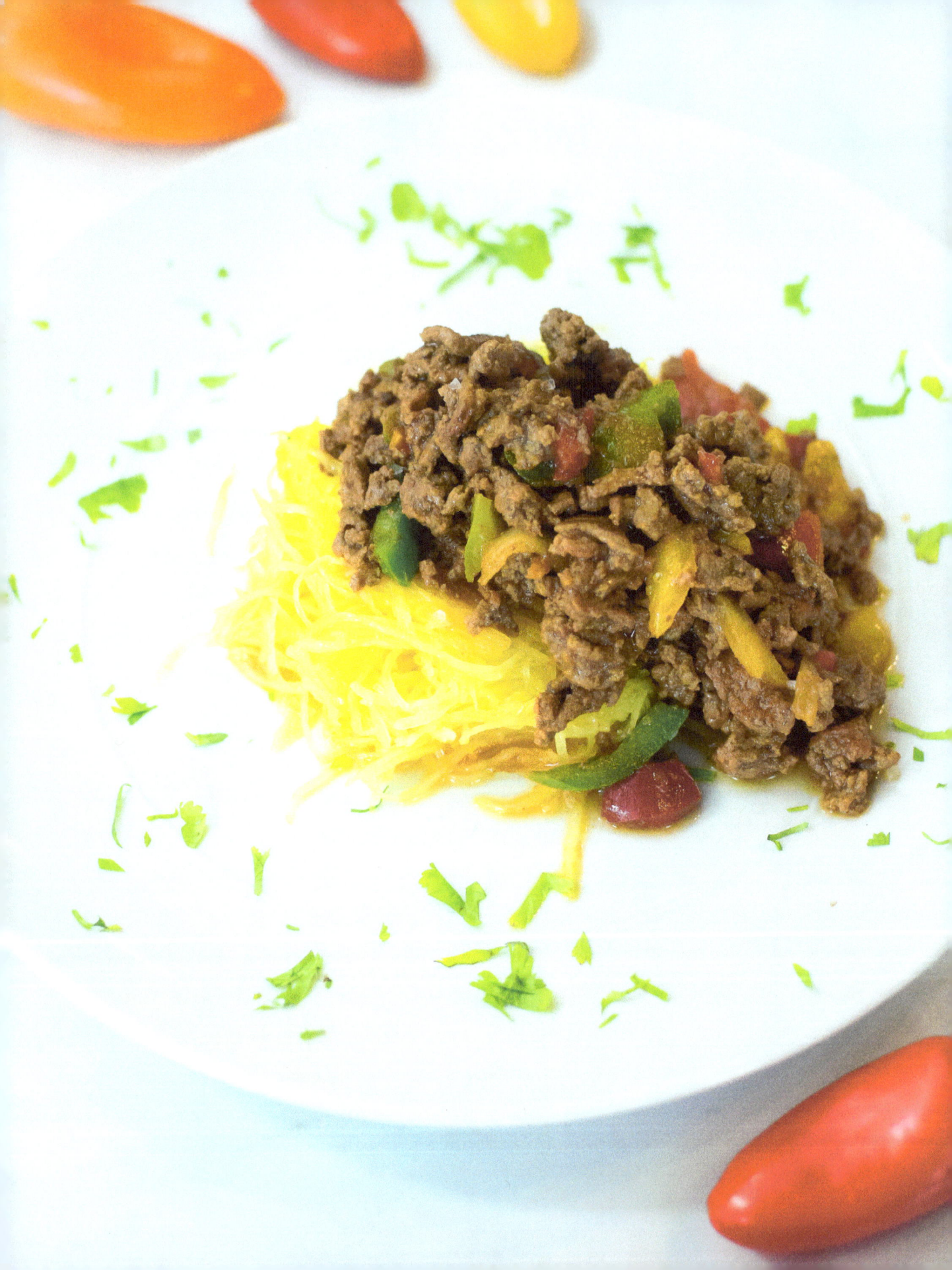

# "DAMN" TURKEY CHILI

Damn this chili is good! Made with earthly vegetables, hearty beans, and ground turkey this will for sure make a delicious dish for a chili winter night. It is also packed with 55 grams of protein to support your appetite and have your "flex on swole like aha, yeah.  Make you feel some type of way then, aha, yeah!" You can also save the left overs for eggs and chili the next day or add it to your Spaghetti Squash and Joe. Hey "don't judge me!"

## Ingredients:

- 1 lb. lean ground turkey
- 1 teaspoon onion powder
- 1 teaspoon garlic powder
- 1 ½ teaspoons of All-Purpose Seasoning with Pepper
- 2 tablespoons olive oil
- 1 cup chopped peppers and onions (fresh or frozen)
- 1 tablespoon chopped garlic
- 1 can tomato sauce
- ½ cup diced tomatoes
- 3 ounces of A1 sauce
- 1 can of navy beans
- Optional: top with cilantro, a squeeze of lime, ½ teaspoon of chili flakes and 1 ounce of shredded mild cheddar cheese

## Directions (makes two servings):

1. Heat oil in a 12" non-stick skillet over medium-high heat.

2. Add chopped onions, peppers, garlic to pan

3. Season ground turkey with Adobo, garlic powder, onion powder and add to pan. Cook until golden brown.

4. Add A1 sauce, tomato sauce, diced tomatoes and ½ cup of water.

5. Open can of navy beans, rinse and add to pan, stir, cover, and cook on low heat for about 5-10 minutes and serve!

## Nutrition Facts

2 servings per container

| Serving size | 8 oz |
|---|---|

**Amount Per Serving**

| Calories | 370 |
|---|---|

| | % Daily Value* |
|---|---|
| **Total Fat** 17g | 22% |
| Saturated Fat 4g | 20% |
| *Trans* Fat 0g | |
| **Cholesterol** 95mg | 32% |
| **Sodium** 770mg | 33% |
| **Total Carbohydrate** 24g | 9% |
| Dietary Fiber 5g | 18% |
| Total Sugars 0g | |
| Includes 0g Added Sugars | 0% |
| **Protein** 29g | 58% |

Not a significant source of vitamin D, calcium, iron, and potassium

* The % Daily Value (DV) tells you how much a nutrient in a serving of food contributes to a daily diet. 2,000 calories a day is used for general nutrition advice.

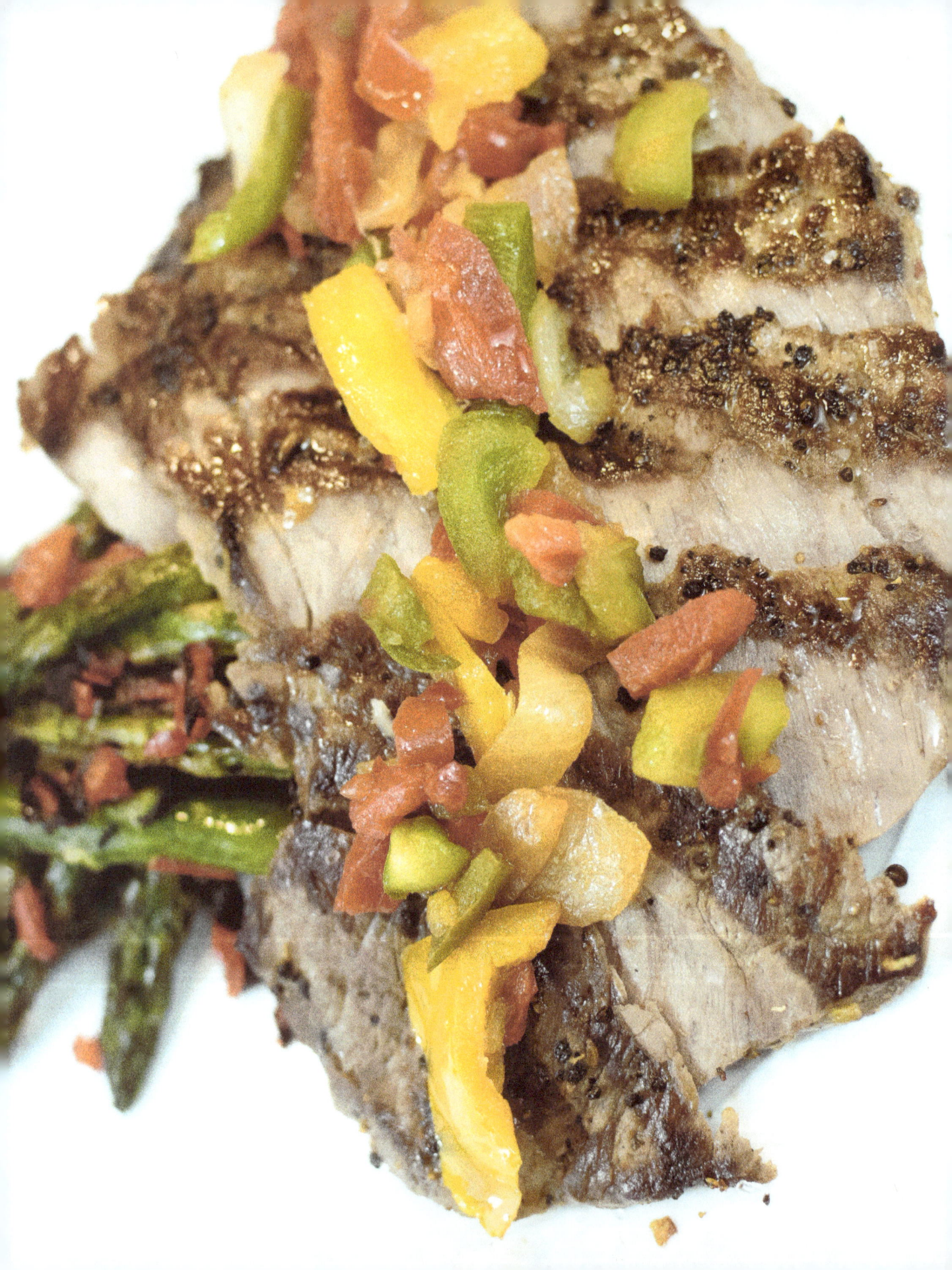

# "FIRE & DESIRE" STEAK & PEPPERS

## Ingredients:

- 6 ounces steak
- ½ cup fresh or frozen peppers
- ½ cup fresh or frozen onions
- 1 teaspoon chopped garlic
- ½ cup fresh or frozen asparagus
- 1 teaspoon sea salt
- Microwaveable Roasted Red Potatoes
- 1 tablespoon Steak Seasoning
- 2 tablespoon olive oil
- Optional: A1 Sauce

Roast your peppers under the fire and grill your steak to your desire! This meal is rich in iron, which is a mineral that transport oxygen to cells throughout the body. Red meats provide a highly absorbable source of iron known as "heme" iron. Dark green vegetables such as asparagus also provide "non-heme" iron to support red blood cell formation. Add the roasted potatoes for a complete meal which provides protein, vegetables, and carbohydrates.

## Directions:

1. Season steak on both sides with McCormick Grill Mates Montreal Steak Seasoning

2. Heat skillet over medium to high heat with oil

3. Add peppers and onions to skillet, cook for 8 min, remove peppers and onions from pan.

4. Season asparagus with sea salt and bake at 400°F

5. Microwave Birds Eye Steamfresh Salt & Vinegar Potatoes for 5 minutes then bake in oven for 10 minutes

6. Cook steak on medium to high heat in the skillet for 6-7 min each side, then add grilled onions and peppers

7. Remove asparagus and potatoes, plate and add steak, enjoy!

## Nutrition Facts

1 servings per container

| Serving size | 1 Steak |
|---|---|

**Amount Per Serving**

| Calories | **830** |
|---|---|

| | % Daily Value* |
|---|---|
| **Total Fat** 48g | **62%** |
| Saturated Fat 12g | **60%** |
| *Trans* Fat 0g | |
| **Cholesterol** 150mg | **50%** |
| **Sodium** 2020mg | **88%** |
| **Total Carbohydrate** 43g | **16%** |
| Dietary Fiber 6g | **21%** |
| Total Sugars 0g | |
| Includes 0g Added Sugars | **0%** |
| **Protein** 55g | **110%** |

Not a significant source of vitamin D, calcium, iron, and potassium

* The % Daily Value (DV) tells you how much a nutrient in a serving of food contributes to a daily diet. 2,000 calories a day is used for general nutrition advice.

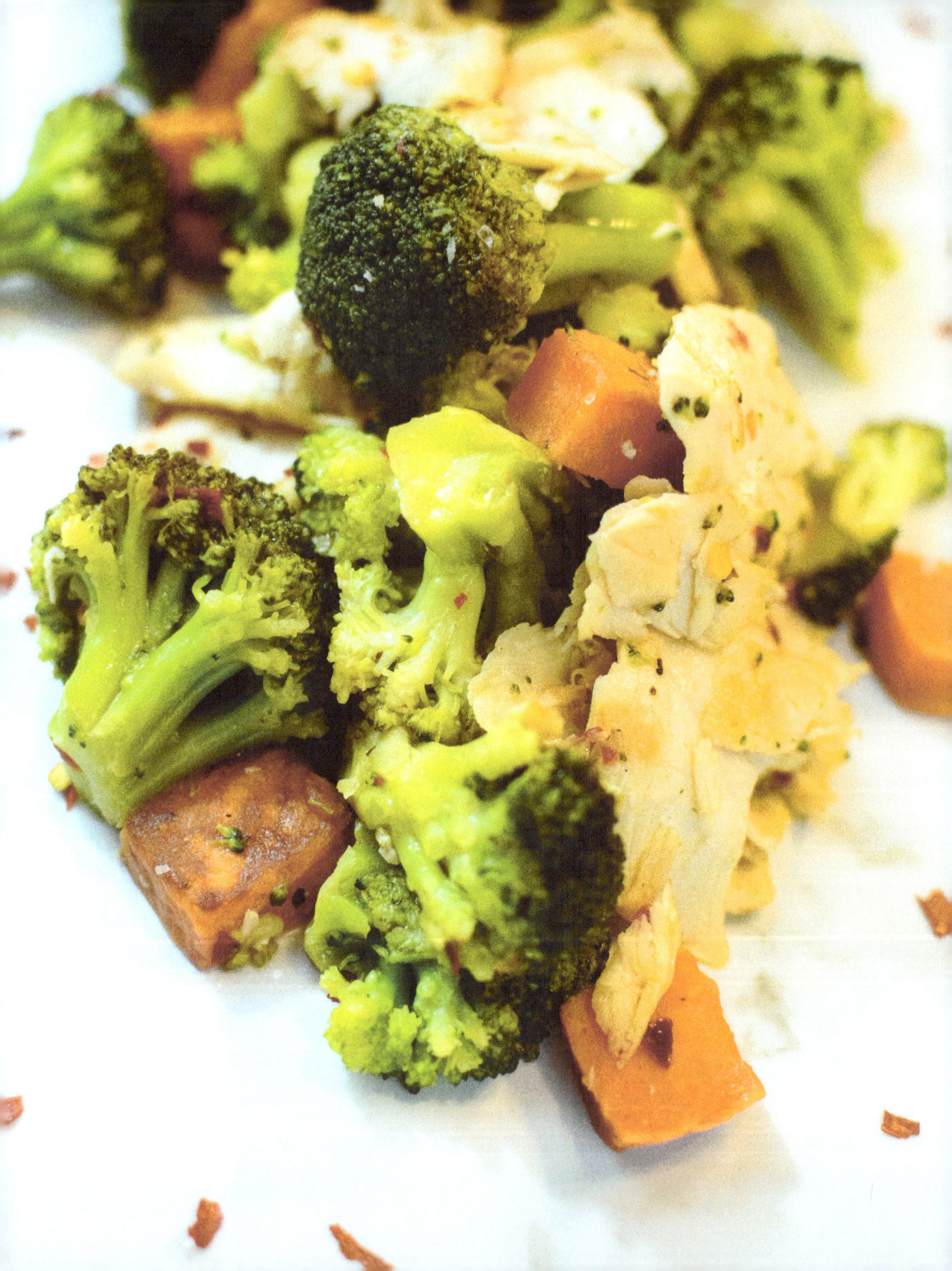

# SWEET CHICKEN AND BROCCOLI

Broccoli is a great source of vitamins K and C; it is also a good source of folate (folic acid) and provides potassium and fiber. Consume broccoli raw, sautéed, boiled or steamed. Cooking broccoli helps to enhance some of the nutritional properties, but if you overcook it the nutritional benefits will be destroyed. Prepare your broccoli to your liking and add a serving of chicken for a complete protein and vegetable rich meal to support health, wellness, and longevity!

## Ingredients:

- 4 ounces of grilled chicken breast
- 1 tablespoon olive oil
- ½ teaspoon salt
- ½ teaspoon pepper
- ½ teaspoon onion powder
- ½ teaspoon garlic powder
- 2 tablespoons butter
- 1 cup of broccoli
- 1 cup of Lightly Seasoned Sweet Potatoes with Brown Sugar

## Directions (makes two servings):

1. Season chicken in bowl with olive oil, salt, pepper, onion powder and garlic powder

2. Heat pan over medium heat with non-stick spray

3. Cook both sides of chicken for 6 min each

4. Microwave the sweet potatoes and broccoli separately for 5 min. each

5. Then heat broccoli in a pan over medium heat with butter

6. Portion out 1 cup of sweet potatoes and 1 cup of broccoli, plate chicken and enjoy!

## Nutrition Facts

1 servings per container

| Serving size | 8 oz |
|---|---|

**Amount Per Serving**

| Calories | 660 |
|---|---|

| | % Daily Value* |
|---|---|
| **Total Fat** 39g | 50% |
| Saturated Fat 9g | 45% |
| *Trans* Fat 0g | |
| **Cholesterol** 95mg | 32% |
| **Sodium** 2020mg | 88% |
| **Total Carbohydrate** 29g | 11% |
| Dietary Fiber 6g | 21% |
| Total Sugars 0g | |
| Includes 0g Added Sugars | 0% |
| **Protein** 42g | 84% |

Not a significant source of vitamin D, calcium, iron, and potassium

* The % Daily Value (DV) tells you how much a nutrient in a serving of food contributes to a daily diet. 2,000 calories a day is used for general nutrition advice.

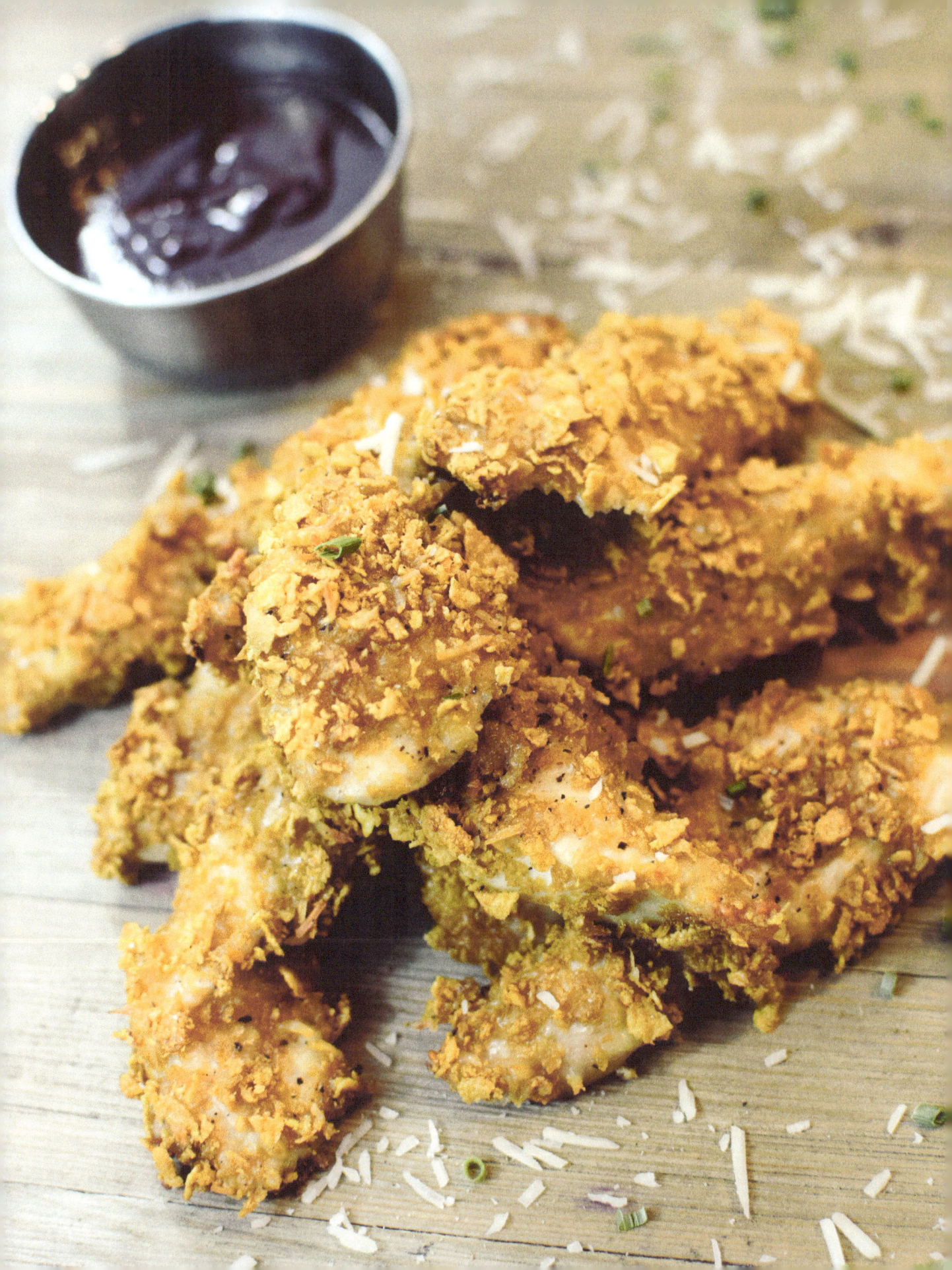

# NAS YOUR AVERAGE FRIED CHICKEN

## Ingredients:

- 4 boneless, skinless chicken breasts
- ¼ cup skim milk
- ½ cup cornflake crumbs
- ¼ cup grated parmesan cheese
- Salt and pepper to taste
- 2 tablespoons olive oil or nonstick spray oil

Fried chicken is a common food in hip-hop culture or any culture for that matter. It can be a delicious dish, but maybe not so nutritious. It will provide plenty of protein, however it is void of vegetables and can often cause excess calorie intake as it is often paired with French fries. Try this modified version of your favorite dish! Not your average fried chicken, but guaranteed to be delicious and more nutritious!

## Directions (makes four servings):

1. Coat bottom of baking pan with spray or oil

2. Combine crumbs and cheese in a bowl

3. Season chicken breasts with salt and pepper

4. Dip chicken into milk, then into crumb mixture

5. Place chicken in dish. Bake at 350°F about 30 minutes, turning every 10 minutes

## Nutrition Facts

1 servings per container

| | |
|---|---|
| **Serving size** | **4 Peices** |

**Amount Per Serving**

**Calories** **230**

| | % Daily Value* |
|---|---|
| **Total Fat** 10g | **13%** |
| Saturated Fat 2g | **10%** |
| *Trans* Fat 0g | |
| **Cholesterol** 70mg | **23%** |
| **Sodium** 650mg | **28%** |
| **Total Carbohydrate** 5g | **2%** |
| Dietary Fiber 0g | **0%** |
| Total Sugars 0g | |
| Includes 0g Added Sugars | **0%** |
| **Protein** 29g | **58%** |

Not a significant source of vitamin D, calcium, iron, and potassium

* The % Daily Value (DV) tells you how much a nutrient in a serving of food contributes to a daily diet. 2,000 calories a day is used for general nutrition advice.

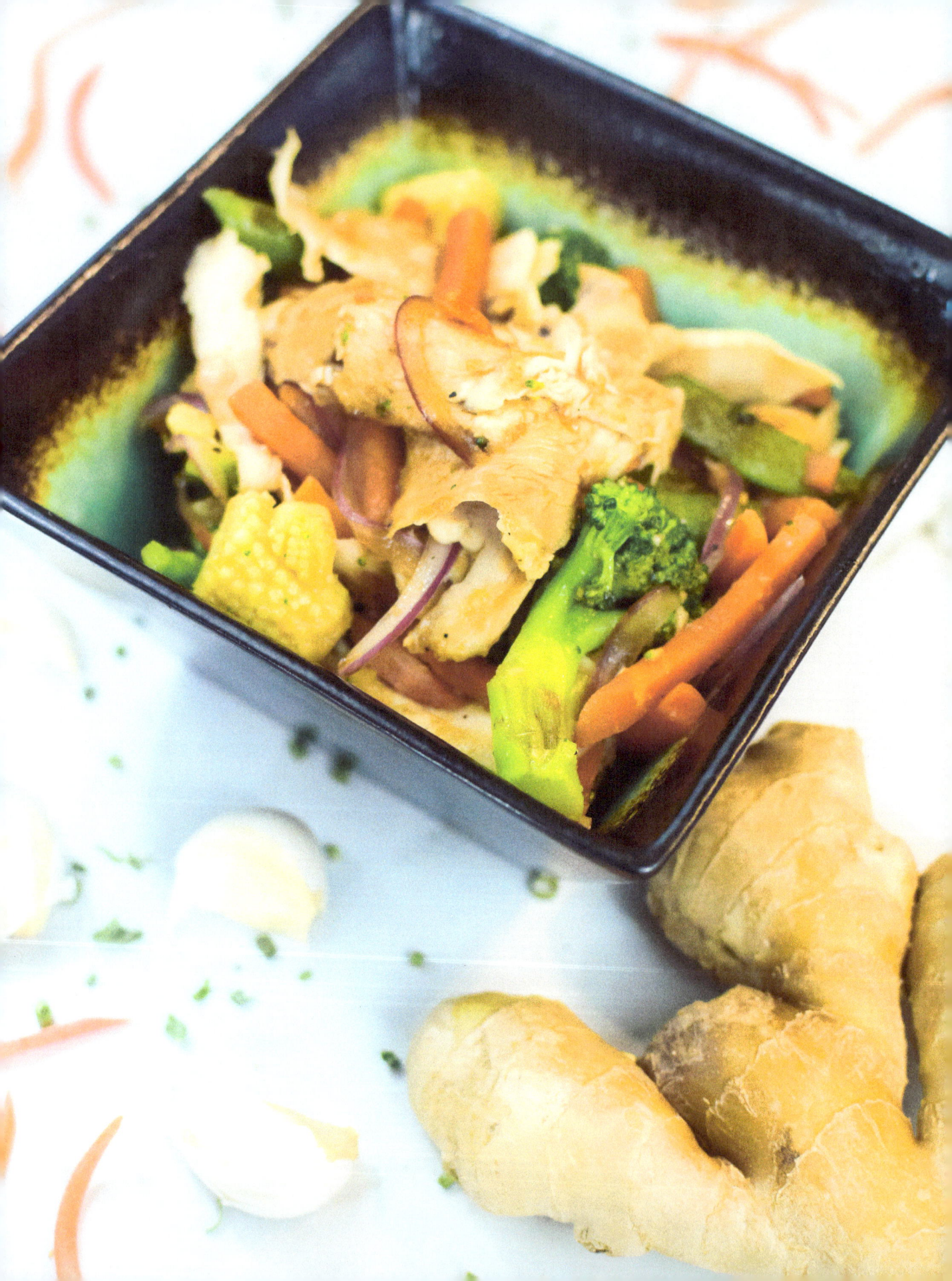

# CHICKEN STIR FRY

Whip up this stir fry in no time! A diverse dish with plenty of carrots, broccoli, snap peas, onions, peppers, water chestnuts, mushrooms, and celery for a mixture of several vitamins and minerals to support your life and vitality! Add grilled chicken for a complete dish!

## Ingredients:

- 4 boneless, skinless chicken breasts
- Birds Eye Recipe Ready Broccoli Stir Fry
- 2 tablespoons ginger paste
- 1 tablespoon soy sauce
- 2 tablespoon honey
- 2 tablespoon olive oil
- 1 ½ teaspoons GOYA Adobo All-Purpose Seasoning with Pepper
- 1 teaspoon pepper
- 1 teaspoon onion powder
- 1 teaspoon garlic powder

## Directions:

1. Cut chicken breasts into short, narrow strips

2. Season chicken with Adobo, pepper, onion powder, ginger paste, and garlic powder

3. In a small bowl mix the soy sauce, and honey together

4. Heat oil in frying pan

5. Add bag of Birds Eye Recipe Ready Broccoli Stir Fry, let cook covered for 5 minutes

6. Add chicken and cook for about 10 minutes

7. Stir occasionally and add the soy sauce and honey mixture

## Nutrition Facts

1 servings per container

| Serving size | 8 oz |
|---|---|

**Amount Per Serving**

**Calories** 200

| | % Daily Value* |
|---|---|
| **Total Fat** 2g | 3% |
| Saturated Fat 0g | 0% |
| *Trans* Fat 0g | |
| **Cholesterol** 65mg | 22% |
| **Sodium** 650mg | 28% |
| **Total Carbohydrate** 17g | 6% |
| Dietary Fiber 2g | 7% |
| Total Sugars 0g | |
| Includes 0g Added Sugars | 0% |
| **Protein** 27g | 54% |

Not a significant source of vitamin D, calcium, iron, and potassium

*The % Daily Value (DV) tells you how much a nutrient in a serving of food contributes to a daily diet. 2,000 calories a day is used for general nutrition advice.

55

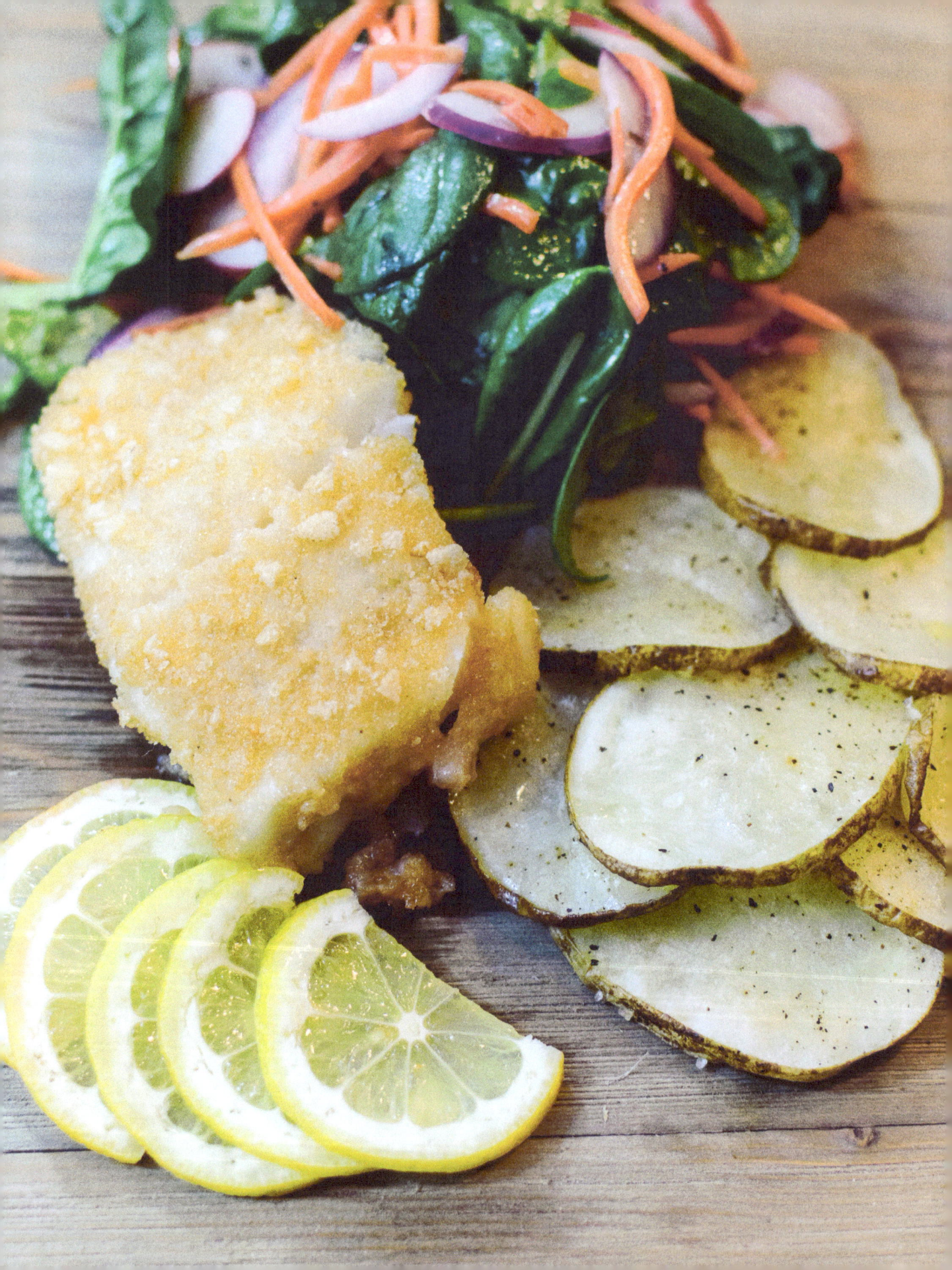

# FINGER LICKING FISH N' CHIPS

## Ingredients:

- 1 lb. fish fillets, cut into sticks
- 2 tablespoons olive or canola oil
- ⅓ cup crispy rice cereal or cornflake crumbs
- 1 whole potato cut into thin slices
- 1 small side salad

Whip up this stir fry in no time! A diverse dish with plenty of carrots, broccoli, snap peas, onions, peppers, water chestnuts, mushrooms, and celery for a mixture of several vitamins and minerals to support your life and vitality! Add grilled chicken for a complete dish!

## Directions:

1. Preheat oven to 450°F.

2. Wash and dry the fish fillets.

3. Season each fillet with sea salt and pepper as desired; coat with oil.

4. Dip the fish fillets into the cereal crumbs .

5. Arrange the fillets on shallow nonstick pan and bake for 12 minutes; don't turn.

6. Cut the whole potato into thin slices and spread on a separate nonstick baking sheet add to oven and cook until golden brown.

7. Serve with a wedge of lemon.

## Nutrition Facts

1 servings per container

| Serving size | 1 Basket |
|---|---|

**Amount Per Serving**

**Calories 630**

| | % Daily Value* |
|---|---|
| **Total Fat** 20g | **26%** |
| Saturated Fat 2g | **10%** |
| *Trans* Fat 0g | |
| **Cholesterol** 100mg | **33%** |
| **Sodium** 3120mg | **136%** |
| **Total Carbohydrate** 62g | **23%** |
| Dietary Fiber 8g | **29%** |
| Total Sugars 0g | |
| Includes 0g Added Sugars | **0%** |
| **Protein** 50g | **100%** |

Not a significant source of vitamin D, calcium, iron, and potassium

*The % Daily Value (DV) tells you how much a nutrient in a serving of food contributes to a daily diet. 2,000 calories a day is used for general nutrition advice.

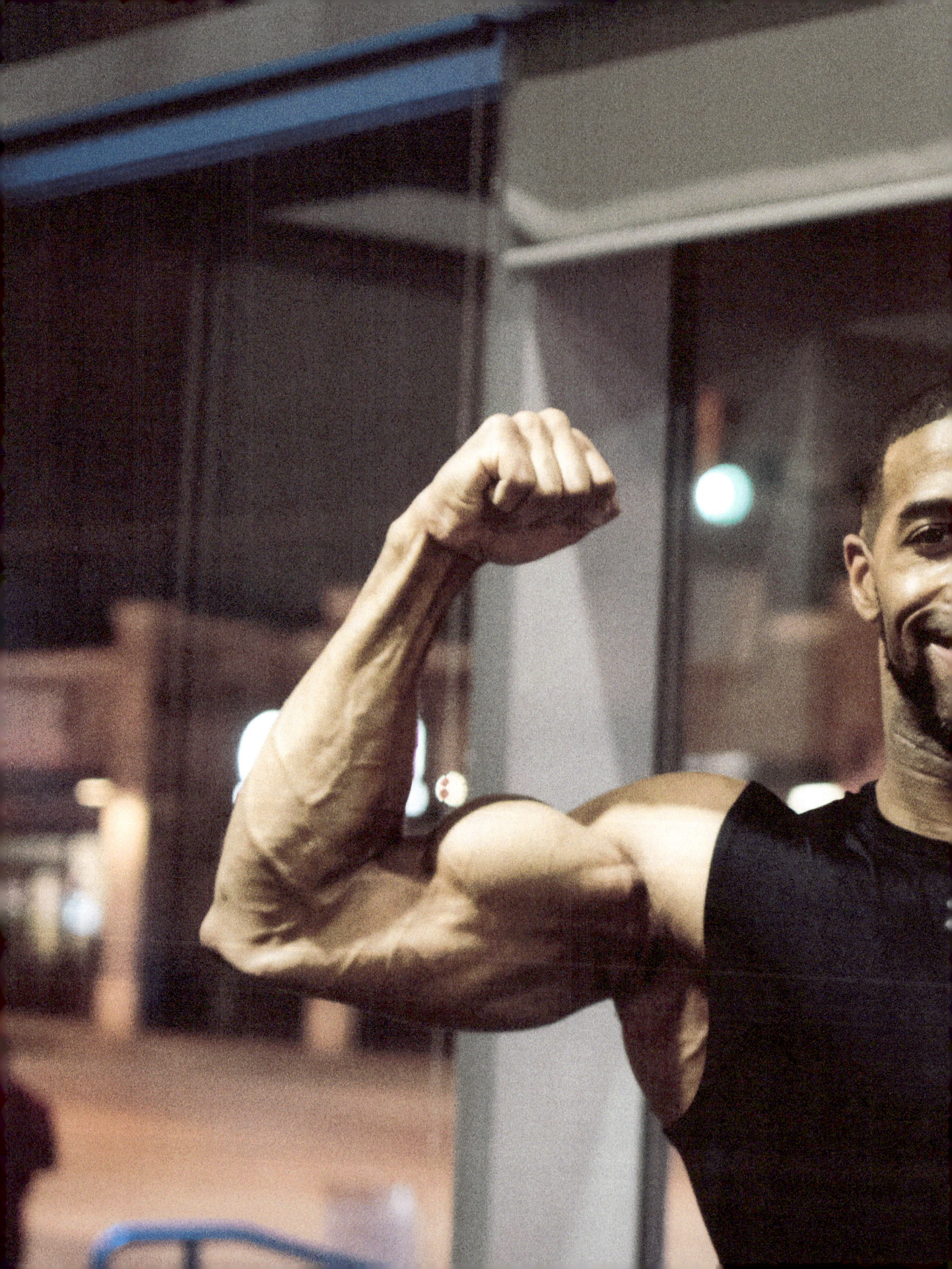

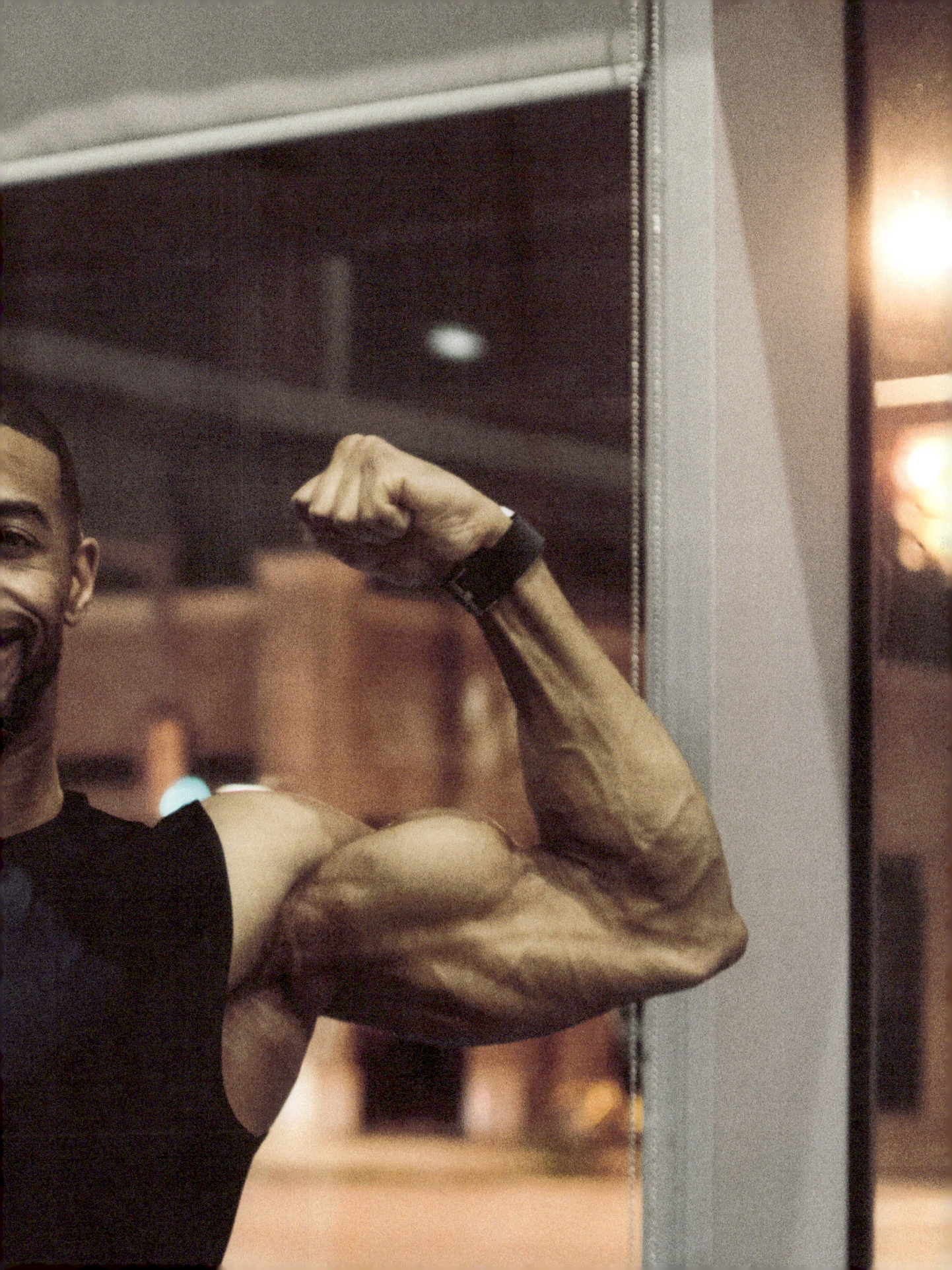

# FRUITS, VEGETABLES, AND PHYTONUTRIENTS TO FIGHT DISEASE

Canned, fresh, frozen, organic, or not, raw, steamed baked or boiled the key is to increase fruit and vegetable intake to extrapolate the phytochemicals, fiber, and anti-oxidants to help fight disease!

**Phytonutrients** – a broad name for a wide variety of compounds produced in plants. They are found in fruits, vegetables, beans, grains, and other plants. Each phytonutrient has a different effect on health and benefit for the body. Researchers estimate that there are up to 4,000 phytonutrients! Only a small fraction has been studied closely!

Common names for phytonutrients – antioxidants, flavonoids, phytochemicals, flavones, isoflavones, catechins, anthocyanidins, isothiocyanates, carotenoids, allyl sulfides, polyphenols.

Antioxidants are one of the most common phytonutrients that we are familiar with. They are substances that prevent (anti) cell damage (oxidation) which helps to prevent diabetes, high blood pressure, heart attacks and even cancer.

| Phytochemical | Proposed Benefits | Food Sources | Fun Facts |
|---|---|---|---|
| Beta-Carotene | Immune System, Vision, Skin Health, Bone Health | Pumpkin, Sweet Potato, Carrots, Cantaloupe, Spinach, Broccoli, Apricots, Greens, Kale | Orange and dark, leafy green veggies |
| Lycopene | Cancer (Prostate), Heart Health | Tomatoes, Pink Grapefruit, Watermelon, Red Peppers | The heating process makes lycopene easier for the body to absorb |
| Lutein | Eye Health, Cancer, Heart Health | Collard Greens, Kale, Spinach, Brussel Sprouts, Broccoli, Lettuces, Artichokes | Found in the macula of the eye |
| Resveratrol | Heart Health, Cancer, Lung Health, Inflammation | Red Wine, Peanuts, Grapes | 1 cup of red grapes can have up to 1.25 mg of resveratrol |
| Anthocyanins | Blood Vessel Health | Blueberries, Blackberries, Strawberries, Plums, Cranberries, Raspberries, Red Onions, Radishes | Think red and purple berries |
| Isoflavones | Menopause, Lower Cholesterol, Bone, Cancer (Breast), Joint, Inflammation | Whole Soybeans | ½ c boiled soybeans provides 47 mg of isoflavones |

Adapted from: https://www.fruitsandveggiesmorematters.org/what-are-phytochemicals

# PROTEIN-RICH FOODS

Protein is necessary to build, maintain, and repair muscle. Proteins are made from amino acids which provide the building blocks for enzymes, hormones, vitamins, bones, muscles, cartilage, skin, and blood. There are nine essential amino acids (EAAs), which are histidine, isoleucine, leucine, lysine, methionine, phenylalanine, threonine, tryptophan, and valine. These EAAs must be provided on a daily basis in the diet in order to allow for optimal muscle-protein synthesis and to minimize muscle protein breakdown overtime. You can obtain a sufficient amount of these essential amino acids by consuming approximately 25 g of total protein for a meal or snack to provide a total of about 10g of EAA. Many foods – including meats, poultry, seafood, eggs, dairy products, beans and nuts contain protein. All EAA are necessary to stimulate muscle protein synthesis.

Lifting weights and eating enough protein at each meal can help to reduce what is known as sarcopenia, or age-related muscle loss. By the age of 40 we can lose 8% of our muscle mass per decade and by age 70 we lose 15% of our muscle per decade. By eating high quality protein foods it allows us to extract all nine essential amino acids which are essential for allowing optimal muscle maintenance or growth if you are resistant exercise training. Aim for 25-35 grams of protein per meal (breakfast, lunch, and dinner) to extract enough EAAs to build and support muscle tissue. A higher protein diet may also help with weight loss by reducing energy intake; improving appetite and controlling hunger and preserving lean body mass. Your protein needs for growth and repair are increased when you work out with weights and place a strain on the muscle tissue. The protein needs following weight baring exercise are essentially higher for the next one to two days.

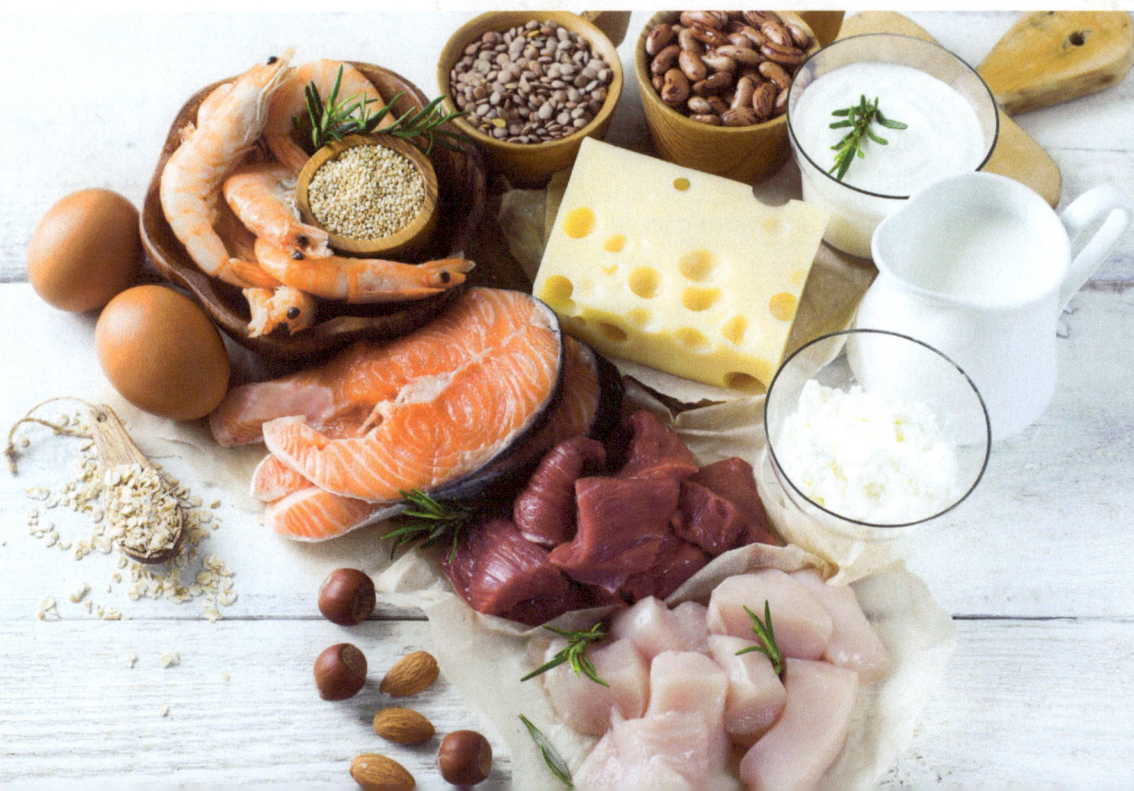

| Food | Portion | Grams of Protein |
|---|---|---|
| Beans, mashed kidney or pinto | ½ cup | 6 |
| Beef, at least 90% lean | 3 ounces | 21 |
| Cheese, low fat | 1 ounce (1 slice) | 6 |
| Cottage cheese, low fat 1% | ½ cup | 14 |
| Cheese, grated parmesan | 2 Tablespoons | 4 |
| Cheese, part skim mozzarella | 1 ounce | 8 |
| Chicken, skinless, white breast meat | 3 ounces | 21 |
| Cod, baked | 3 ounces | 21 |
| Edamame, cooked | 3.5 ounces | 12 |
| Egg, hard boiled | 1 | 7 |
| Egg, whites | 2 | 7 |
| Egg substitute | ½ cup | 12 |
| Flounder, baked | 3 ounces | 21 |
| Halibut, baked | 3 ounces | 21 |
| Ham, lean 5% fat | 3 ounces | 21 |
| Kefir | 8 ounces | 10 |
| Lobster, steamed | 3 ounces | 16 |
| Milk, skim* | 1 cup | 8 |
| Milk, skim plus | 1 cup | 11 |
| Pork loin chop | 3 ounces | 21 |
| Peanut butter, reduced fat | 2 Tablespoons | 8 |
| Salmon, baked* | 3 ounces | 21 |
| Sardines, in water | 1 can | 23 |
| Shrimp, medium, cooked | 3 ounces | 17 |
| Swordfish, baked | 3 ounces | 21 |
| Soy milk | 1cup | 11 |
| Tofu, firm raw | ½ cup | 20 |
| Tuna, canned and water packed | 3 ounces | 25 |
| Turkey, white meat | 3 ounces | 21 |
| Yogurt, fat free and no sugar added | 4 ounces | 6 |
| Yogurt, Greek, any flavor | 5.3 ounces | 14.5 |

# OMEGA-3 FATTY ACID RICH FOODS

Omega 3 fatty acids are made up of eicosapentaenoic acid (EPA) and docosahexaenoic acid (DHA) which are essential fatty acids, meaning that they are essential for life functions such as supporting the brain and nervous system and they also must be obtained from the diet. Omega 3 fatty acids may also be beneficial for blood pressure, immunity, and reducing systemic inflammation. The omega-3 content of fish varies widely. Cold-water fatty fish, such as salmon, mackerel, tuna, herring, and sardines, contain high amounts of omega-3 content, whereas fish such as bass, tilapia and cod-as well as shellfish contain lower levels. There are plant oils that contain omega-3 fatty acids as well, but primarily in the form of alpha-linolenic acid (ALA) which can then be converted to EPA and DHA in the liver, however this process occurs at a very limited rate. Flaxseeds, soybeans, walnuts, chia seed and canola oils are rich in ALA, but contain very little to no DHA and EPA. Aim for 250-500 mg of omega 3 fatty acids per day.

With respect to seafood and omega-3s, the Dietary Guidelines for Americans state that:

"Strong evidence from mostly prospective cohort studies but also randomized controlled trials has shown that eating patterns that include seafood are associated with reduced risk of cardiovascular disease (CVD), and moderate evidence indicates that these eating patterns are associated with reduced risk of obesity."

"For the general population, consumption of about 8 ounces per week of a variety of seafood, which provide an average consumption of 250 mg per day of EPA and DHA, is associated with reduced cardiac deaths among individuals with and without preexisting CVD."

"Similarly, consumption by women who are pregnant or breastfeeding of at least 8 ounces per week from seafood choices that are sources of DHA is associated with improved infant health outcomes."

"Women who are pregnant or breastfeeding should consume at least 8 and up to 12 ounces of a variety of seafood per week, from choices that are lower in methyl mercury."

63

For more information about building a healthy diet, refer to the Dietary Guidelines for Americans and the U.S. Department of Agriculture's MyPlate.

## Selected Food Sources of ALA, EPA, and DHA

| Food | ALA mg/serving | DHA mg/serving | EPA mg/servings |
|---|---|---|---|
| Salmon, Atlantic, farmed cooked, 3 ounces | 0 mg | 1,2400 mg | 590 mg |
| Salmon, Atlantic, wild, cooked, 3 ounces | 0 mg | 1,220 mg | 350 mg |
| Herring, Atlantic, cooked, 3 ounces * | 0 mg | 940 mg | 770 mg |
| Canola oil, 1 tbsp | 1,280 mg | 0 mg | 0 mg |
| Sardines, canned in tomato sauce, drained, 3 ounces* | 0 mg | 740 mg | 450 mg |
| Mackerel, Atlantic, cooked, 3 ounces* | 0 mg | 590 mg | 430 mg |
| Salmon, pink, canned, drained, 3 ounces* | 40 mg | 630 mg | 280 mg |
| Trout, rainbow, wild, cooked, 3 ounces | 0 mg | 440 mg | 400 mg |
| Black walnuts, 1 ounce | 760 mg | 0 | 0 |
| Oysters, eastern, wild, cooked, 3 ounces | 140 mg | 230 mg | 300 mg |
| Sea bass, cooked, 3 ounces* | 0 mg | 470 mg | 180 mg |
| Shrimp, cooked, 3 ounces* | 0 mg | 120 mg | 120 mg |
| Lobster, cooked, 3 ounces* | 40 mg | 70 mg | 100 mg |
| Tuna, light, canned in water, drained, 3 ounces* | 0 mg | 170 mg | 20 mg |
| Tilapia, cooked, 3 ounces* | 40 mg | 110 mg | 0 |
| Cod, Pacific, cooked, 3 ounces* | 0 mg | 100 mg | 40 mg |
| Tuna, yellowfin, cooked 3 ounces* | 0 mg | 90 mg | 10 mg |

For a supplemental source of Omega 3 fatty acids try CoroMega Max Fish Oil. Coromega Max has a powerful 2,400mg of Omega-3 fatty acids including DHA+EPA which means the maximum health benefits for the heart, body and mind. Our delicious coconut bliss formula is uniquely emulsified to provide 300% better absorption than standard soft gels. Coromega Max delivers the optimum omega-3 for the elite athlete in all of us.

Use code **James7** for $7 off!

https://www.maxfishoil.com/

Adapted from: https://ods.od.nih.gov/factsheets/Omega3FattyAcids-HealthProfessional/#en29 Table 2 Selected Food Sources of ALA, EPA, and DHA. U.S. Department of Agriculture, Agricultural Research Service. USDA National Nutrient Database for Standard Reference, Release 28. external link disclaimer Nutrient Data Laboratory Home Page, 2015.

*Except as noted, the USDA database does not specify whether fish are farmed or wild caught.

# VITAMINS AND MINERALS

First, it is important to know that a multivitamin does not replace a healthy, well balanced diet. It is best to eat a well-balanced diet to obtain the necessary number of vitamins and minerals to support life. Multivitamins and minerals do not appear to reduce overall chronic disease risk, several nutrients in multivitamins might benefit certain population groups such as supplementing with calcium and vitamin D for postmenopausal women; women of childbearing age who are trying to become pregnant should obtain 40 mcg/day of synthetic folic acid from fortified foods or dietary supplements; people over the age of 50 and vegans should obtain the recommended amount of vitamin B12, calcium and vitamin D from foods or supplements; pregnant women should consider an iron supplement as recommended by an obstetrician or other healthcare provider. Those who have undergone bariatric surgery, people with certain diseases such as Celiac or Crohn's disease may have risk for nutrient deficiencies due to poor absorption.

The American Academy of Pediatrics recommends that exclusively and partially breastfed infants receive 400 IU/day of vitamin D. Individuals with poor nutrients intakes from diet alone, who consume low calorie diets, or who avoid certain foods (such as strict vegetarians and vegans) might benefit from taking a multivitamin. Check out the chart below to find out more about vitamins and minerals; what it does, where it is found in foods and what the recommended daily value is.

| Vitamin | What it does | Where is it found | Daily Value* |
|---|---|---|---|
| Biotin | • Energy storage<br>• Protein, carbohydrate, and fat metabolism | • Avocados<br>• Cauliflower<br>• Eggs<br>• Fruits (e.g., raspberries)<br>• Liver<br>• Pork<br>• Salmon<br>• Whole grains | 300 mcg/ day |
| Folate/ Folic Acid | • Important for pregnant women and women capable of becoming pregnant<br>• Prevention of birth defects<br>• Protein metabolism<br>• Red blood cell formation | • Asparagus<br>• Avocado<br>• Beans and peas<br>• Enriched grain products (e.g., bread, cereal, pasta, rice)<br>• Green leafy vegetables (e.g., spinach)<br>• Orange juice | 400 mcg/ day |

| Vitamin | What it does | Where is it found | Daily Value* |
|---|---|---|---|
| Pantothenic Acid | • Conversion of food into energy<br>• Fat metabolism<br>• Hormone production<br>• Nervous system function<br>• Red blood cell formation | • Avocados<br>• Beans and peas<br>• Broccoli<br>• Eggs<br>• Milk<br>• Mushrooms<br>• Poultry<br>• Seafood<br>• Sweet potatoes<br>• Whole grains<br>• Yogurt | 10 mg/ day |
| Niacin | • Cholesterol production<br>• Conversion of food into energy<br>• Digestion<br>• Nervous system function | • Beans<br>• Beef<br>• Enriched grain products (e.g., bread, cereal, pasta, rice)<br>• Nuts<br>• Pork<br>• Poultry<br>• Seafood<br>• Whole grains | 20 mg/ day |
| Riboflavin | • Conversion of food into energy<br>• Growth and development<br>• Red blood cell formation | • Eggs<br>• Enriched grain products (e.g., bread, cereal, pasta, rice)<br>• Meats<br>• Milk<br>• Mushrooms<br>• Poultry<br>• Seafood (e.g., oysters)<br>• Spinach | 1.7 mg/day |
| Thiamin | • Conversion of food into energy<br>• Nervous system function | • Beans and peas<br>• Enriched grain products (e.g., bread, cereal, pasta, rice)<br>• Nuts<br>• Pork<br>• Sunflower seeds<br>• Whole grains | 1.1 mg/ day |

| Vitamin | What it does | Where is it found | Daily Value* |
|---|---|---|---|
| Vitamin A | • Growth and development<br>• Immune function<br>• Reproduction<br>• Red blood cell formation<br>• Skin and bone formation<br>• Vision | • Cantaloupe<br>• Carrots<br>• Dairy products<br>• Eggs<br>• Fortified cereals<br>• Green leafy vegetables (e.g., spinach and broccoli)<br>• Pumpkin<br>• Red peppers<br>• Sweet potatoes | 5,000 IU/ day |
| Vitamin B6 | • Immune function<br>• Nervous system function<br>• Protein, Carbohydrate, and fat metabolism<br>• Red blood cell formation | • Chickpeas<br>• Fruits (other than citrus)<br>• Potatoes<br>• Salmon<br>• Tuna | 2 mg / day |
| Vitamin B12 | • Conversion of food into energy<br>• Nervous system function<br>• Red blood cell formation | • Dairy products<br>• Eggs<br>• Fortified cereals<br>• Meats<br>• Poultry<br>• Seafood (e.g., clams, trout, salmon, haddock, tuna) | 46 mcg /day |
| Vitamin C | • Antioxidant<br>• Collagen and connective tissue formation<br>• Immune function<br>• Wound healing | • Broccoli<br>• Brussel sprouts<br>• Cantaloupe<br>• Citrus fruits and juices (e.g., oranges and grapefruit)<br>• Kiwifruit<br>• Peppers<br>• Strawberries<br>• Tomatoes & tomato juice | 60 mg / day |
| Vitamin D (Nutrient of concern for most Americans) | • Blood pressure regulation<br>• Bone growth<br>• Calcium balance<br>• Hormone production<br>• Immune function<br>• Nervous system function | • Eggs<br>• Fish (e.g., herring, mackerel, salmon, trout, and tuna)<br>• Fish liver oil<br>• Fortified cereals<br>• Fortified dairy products<br>• Fortified margarine<br>• Fortified orange juice<br>• Fortified soy beverages (soymilk) | 400 IU / day |

| Vitamin | What it does | Where is it found | Daily Value* |
|---------|-------------|-------------------|--------------|
| Vitamin E | • Antioxidant<br>• Formation of blood vessels<br>• Immune function | • Fortified cereals and juice<br>• Green vegetables (e.g., spinach and broccoli)<br>• Nuts and seeds<br>• Peanuts and peanut butter<br>• Vegetable oils | 30 IU / day |
| Vitamin K | • Blood clotting<br>• Strong bones | • Green vegetables (e.g., broccoli, kale, spinach, turnip greens, collards, Swiss chard, mustard greens) | 80 mcg / day |

\* - The Daily Values are the amounts of nutrients recommended per day for Americans 4 years of age or older.

| Mineral | What it does | Where is it found | Daily Value* |
|---------|-------------|-------------------|--------------|
| Calcium (Nutrient of concern for most Americans) | • Blood clotting<br>• Bone and teeth formation<br>• Constriction and relaxation of blood vessels<br>• Hormone secretion<br>• Muscle contraction<br>• Nervous system function | • Almond, rice, coconut, and hemp milks<br>• Canned seafood with bones (e.g., salmon and sardines)<br>• Dairy products<br>• Fortified cereals and juices<br>• Fortified soy beverages (soymilk)<br>• Green vegetables (e.g., spinach, kale, broccoli, turnip greens)<br>• Tofu (made with calcium sulfate) | 1000 mg/ day |
| Chloride | • Acid-base balance<br>• Conversion of food into energy<br>• Digestion<br>• Fluid balance<br>• Nervous system function | • Celery<br>• Lettuce<br>• Olives<br>• Rye<br>• Salt substitutes<br>• Seaweeds (e.g., dulse and kelp)<br>• Table salt and sea salt<br>• Tomatoes | 3,400 mg |

| Mineral | What it does | Where is it found | Daily Value* |
|---|---|---|---|
| Chromium | • Insulin function<br>• Protein, carbohydrate, and fat metabolism | • Broccoli<br>• Fruits (e.g., apple and banana)<br>• Grape and orange juice<br>• Meats<br>• Spices (e.g., garlic and basil)<br>• Turkey<br>• Whole grains | 120 mcg / day |
| Copper | • Antioxidant<br>• Bone formation<br>• Collagen and connective tissue formation<br>• Energy production<br>• Iron metabolism<br>• Nervous system function | • Chocolate and cocoa<br>• Crustaceans and shellfish<br>• Lentils<br>• Nuts and seeds<br>• Organ meats (e.g., liver)<br>• Whole grains | 2 mg / day |
| Iodine | • Growth and development<br>• Metabolism<br>• Reproduction<br>• Thyroid hormone production | • Breads and cereals<br>• Dairy products<br>• Iodized salt<br>• Potatoes<br>• Seafood<br>• Seaweed<br>• Turkey | 150 mcg / day |
| Iron (Nutrient of concern for young children, pregnant women, and women capable of becoming pregnant) | • Energy production<br>• Growth and development<br>• Immune function<br>• Red blood cell formation<br>• Reproduction<br>• Wound healing | • Beans and peas<br>• Dark green vegetables<br>• Meats<br>• Poultry<br>• Prunes and prune juice<br>• Raisins<br>• Seafood<br>• Whole grain, enriched, and fortified cereals and breads | 18 mg / day |
| Magnesium | • Blood pressure regulation<br>• Blood sugar regulation<br>• Bone formation<br>• Energy production<br>• Hormone secretion<br>• Immune function<br>• Muscle contraction<br>• Nervous system function<br>• Normal heart rhythm<br>• Protein formation | • Avocados<br>• Bananas<br>• Beans and peas<br>• Dairy products<br>• Green leafy vegetables (e.g., spinach)<br>• Nuts and pumpkin seeds<br>• Potatoes<br>• Raisins<br>• Wheat bran<br>• Whole grains | 400 mg / day |

| Mineral | What it does | Where is it found | Daily Value* |
|---|---|---|---|
| Manganese | • Carbohydrate, protein, and cholesterol metabolism<br>• Cartilage and bone formation<br>• Wound healing | • Beans<br>• Nuts<br>• Pineapple<br>• Spinach<br>• Sweet potato<br>• Whole grains | 2 mg / day |
| Molybdenum | • Enzyme production | • Beans and peas<br>• Nuts<br>• Whole grains | 75 mcg/ day |
| Phosphorus | • Acid-base balance<br>• Bone formation<br>• Energy production and storage<br>• Hormone activation | • Beans and peas<br>• Dairy products<br>• Meats<br>• Nuts and seeds<br>• Poultry<br>• Seafood<br>• Whole grain, enriched, and fortified cereals and breads | 1,000 mg / day |
| Potassium (Nutrient of concern for most Americans) | • Blood pressure regulation<br>• Carbohydrate metabolism<br>• Fluid balance<br>• Growth and development<br>• Heart function<br>• Muscle contraction<br>• Nervous system function<br>• Protein formation | • Bananas<br>• Beet greens<br>• Juices (e.g., carrot, pomegranate, prune, orange, and tomato)<br>• Milk<br>• Oranges and orange juice<br>• Potatoes & sweet potatoes<br>• Prunes and prune juice<br>• Spinach<br>• Tomatoes & tomato products<br>• White beans<br>• Yogurt | 3,500, g/ day |
| Selenium | • Antioxidant<br>• Immune function<br>• Reproduction<br>• Thyroid function | • Eggs<br>• Enriched pasta and rice<br>• Meats<br>• Nuts (e.g., Brazil nuts) & seeds<br>• Poultry<br>• Seafood<br>• Whole grains | 70 mcg/ day |

| Mineral | What it does | Where is it found | Daily Value* |
|---------|-------------|-------------------|--------------|
| Sodium (Nutrient to get less of) | <ul><li>Acid-base balance</li><li>Blood pressure regulation</li><li>Fluid balance</li><li>Muscle contraction</li><li>Nervous system function</li></ul> | <ul><li>Breads and rolls</li><li>Cheese (natural and processed)</li><li>Cold cuts and cured meats (e.g., deli or packaged ham or turkey)</li><li>Mixed pasta dishes (e.g., lasagna, pasta salad, and spaghetti with meat sauce)</li><li>Pizza</li><li>Poultry (fresh and processed)</li><li>Sandwiches (e.g. hamburgers, hot dogs, and submarine sandwiches)</li><li>Savory snacks (e.g. chips, crackers, popcorn, and pretzels)</li><li>Soups</li><li>Table salt</li></ul> | 2,400 mg / day |
| Zinc | <ul><li>Growth and development</li><li>Immune function</li><li>Nervous system function</li><li>Protein formation</li><li>Reproduction</li><li>Taste and smell</li><li>Wound healing</li></ul> | <ul><li>Beans and peas</li><li>Beef</li><li>Dairy products</li><li>Fortified cereals</li><li>Nuts</li><li>Poultry</li><li>Seafood (e.g. clams, crabs, lobsters, oysters)</li><li>Whole grains</li></ul> | |

# Vitamins and Minerals to Consider Supplementing

If you are eating a well-balanced diet you likely will not need a multivitamin. However, there are certain vitamins and minerals which may be needed for supplementation under certain conditions and circumstances, particularly if you're not eating a well-balanced diet. Check with you doctor or consult with a dietitian to find out what nutrients you may be deficient in that you may require supplementation.

**MULTIVITAMINS FOR VEGETARIANS:**

- Calcium and Vitamin D – bone health, immune function, inflammatory modulation, skeletal muscle function. All individuals should consider supplementing with 1000 IU of vitamin D especially in the winter months.

- Iron – red blood cells, oxygen transport, risk for anemia, heme vs non-heme

- Zinc – reduced availability in plant vs. animal foods, high phytic acid in plant foods

- Iodine – excluding consumption of plant foods grown in soil low in iodine, limited cow's milk, fish, or sea products

- Vitamin B12 – cobalamin the active form of vitamin B12 is found exclusively in animal products

- Riboflavin – may be low in those who avoid dairy products

**MICRONUTRIENTS TO CONSIDER FOR THOSE FOLLOWING A "GLUTEN-FREE" DIET:**

The potential cause of deficiency may be related to avoiding wheat products which eliminates some of the nutrients found in those foods, careful dietary planning with nutritious gluten-free foods and choosing fortified rice products may help to reduce risk for deficiency. Main nutrients of concern:

- Calcium
- Iron
- Magnesium
- Zonce
- Folate
- Thiamin
- Vitamin B12
- Vitamin D

**MICRONUTRIENTS TO CONSIDER FOR THOSE FOLLOWING A "LOW-CARB" DIET:**

When following a low-carb diet you have to be mindful of your food choices and what food groups you may be eliminating (i.e. fruits) which may cause deficiencies in your diet. If you are following a low carb diet you should focus on low-carbohydrate vegetables and nuts. Main nutrients of concern:

- Calcium
- Copper
- Magnesium
- Potassium
- Pantothenic acid
- Vitamin E

## MICRONUTRIENTS TO CONSIDER FOR THOSE FOLLOWING A "PALEO" DIET:

When following a Paleo diet you are primarily restricting dairy and legumes. You may be able to counter the nutrient deficits associated with following this restrictive diet by including more leafy greens and nuts. Main nutrients of concern:

- Calcium
- Iodine
- Riboflavin
- Thiamin

Core Health Products has a line of great whole fruit and vegetable based vitamins & minerals. Order your Core Health multivitamins here:

# INSIDETRACKER

You don't really know if you need to supplement with individual nutrients until you have had a dietary analysis or lab parameters assessed to check if you may have any signs or symptoms of nutrient deficiencies. There is no one perfect diet, we make daily adjustments based upon our appetite, activity level and the foods available around us. Changes in our biochemistry occur over days, weeks, months and years. Striving to maintain an optimal diet based upon what you know as good is the key to longevity, however we can take advantage of today's technology and have a full panel blood analysis done to see if we may have deficiencies or imbalances. And even at this point there is still room for improvement and the unknowns, but at least you can put a finger on an issue that would otherwise spiral out of control, causing potential long term disease risk and suboptimal performance on a day to day basis. This is why I have been recommending Inside Tracker for several years, for those who want to take it another step beyond the diet recall to assess for potential metabolic imbalances. Have an Inside Tracker test done today.

> "What if you could take a selfie... from the inside" Learn what you need. Make changes. Feel better, perform your best.
>
> Inside Tracker

www.insidetracker.com

Use code JamesLucas10 to save 10% off your order!

## Ultimate $589
*Take control of your destiny*
- 42 Total Biomarkers
- InnerAge Upgradeable

Order Now ▸
View Details ▸

Raise metabolism · Improve cognition · Maintain bone health · Enhance performance
Build muscle · Aid liver function · Reduce inflammation · Boost energy · Optimize mood

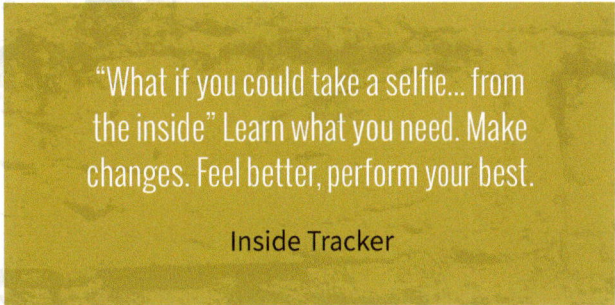

2 tests SAVE $189
4 tests SAVE $657

## Vitality $389
*Get the Competitive Edge*
- 19 Total Biomarkers
- Perfect for the Weekend Warrior or Serious Athlete

Order Now ▸
View Details ▸

Improve cognition · Maintain bone health · Enhance performance
Reduce inflammation · Raise metabolism · Optimize mood

2 tests SAVE $100
4 tests SAVE $297

## High Performance $299
*Push your performance past its peak*
- 11 Biomarkers

Order Now ▸
View Details ▸

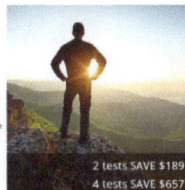

Enhance performance · Reduce inflammation · Improve cognition · Maintain bone health · Aid liver function

2 tests SAVE $79
4 tests SAVE $240

## Essentials $189
*Improve your Body and Mind*
- 12 Total Biomarkers
- Design and Protect The Body You Want

Order Now ▸
View Details ▸

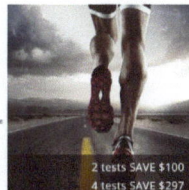

Raise metabolism · Maintain bone health · Enhance performance

2 tests SAVE $38
4 tests SAVE $114

## InnerAge $99
*Gain Life and Vitality*
- 5 Key Biomarkers for Life
- Calculate Your Real Age from the Inside

Order Now ▸
View Details ▸

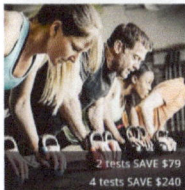

InnerAge

2 tests SAVE $19
4 tests SAVE $57

## Home kit starting from $109
*Increase Wellness Anywhere*
- 7 Wellness Biomarkers
- Maintain an Active Lifestyle from Home

Order Now ▸
View Details ▸

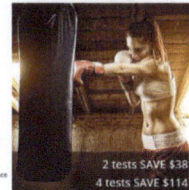

Reduce inflammation · Raise metabolism · Boost energy

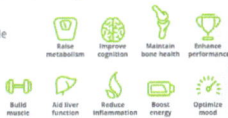
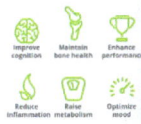
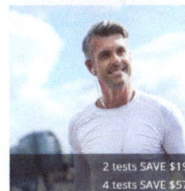
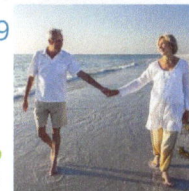

# FRUITS, VEGETABLES & PLANT-BASED FOODS FOR CANCER PREVENTION

*"Let food be thy medicine and medicine be thy food."*

**HIPPOCRATES**

| FOODS | PHYTOCHEMICALS | VITAMINS | FIBER | ANTIOXIDANT ACTIVITY | STIMULATES ANTICANCER ENZYMES | ACTS AS CANCER INHIBITOR |
|---|---|---|---|---|---|---|
| Garlic; onion (Allium vegetables) | Organosulfur compounds | | Soluble, insoluble | X | | X |
| Broccoli, cauliflower, cabbage, and other cruciferous vegetables (Brassica) vegetables | Indoles, sulforaphane, isothiocynate | Folate, vitamins A and C | Insoluble | | | X |
| Citrus fruit | Terpenes, coumarins, flavonoids | Vitamin C, folate | Soluble | X | X | X |
| Strawberries, grapes, apples, berries, and nuts | Ellagic acid | Vitamins E & C, beta carotene | Soluble | X | X | X |
| Carrots, yams, cantaloupe, butternut squash | | Beta carotene | Soluble, insoluble | X | X | X |
| Soybeans, beans, peas, lentils | Genistein, other isoflavones, saponins, phytosterols | | Soluble | | | X |
| Hot peppers | Capsaicin | Vitamin C | | X | | X |
| Flaxseed, whole wheat, barley, brown rice | Lignans | | Soluble, insoluble | X | | X |
| Tomatoes, red grapefruit | Lycopene | Vitamin C | Soluble | X | | X |
| Green tea, grapes | Polyphenols | | | | | X |

# METRIC CONVERSIONS

## English (U.S.) to Metric
Pounds x 0.454 = kilograms
Ounces x 28.35 = grams
Quarts x 0.946 = liters
Cups x 236.6 = milliliters
Inches x 2.5 = centimeters

## Metric to English (U.S.)
Kilograms x 2.2 = pounds
Grams x 0.035 = ounces
Liters x 1.056 = quarts
Cups x 236.6 = milliliters
Centimeters = 0.4 inches

## Common Measurements Used in Food
3 t = 1 T
12 T = ¾ c
4 c = 1 qt.
16 T = 1 c
5 ⅓ T = ⅓ c
4 qts. = 1 gal
4 T = ¼ c
10 ⅔ T = ⅔ c
2 T = 1 liquid oz.
8 T = ½ c
2 c = 1 pt.
8 oz. = 1 c or ½ pt.

## Metric Measurement

| Volume | Approximate Weight |
|--------|--------------------|
| 160ml | 140g |
| 120ml | 110g |
| 90ml | 85-100g |
| 80ml | 70-85g |
| 60ml | 60-70g |
| 45ml | 50g |
| 40ml | 40g |
| 30ml | 30g |
| 24ml | 23g |
| 15ml | 15g |

## English Measurement (U.S.)

| Volume | Approximate Weight |
|--------|--------------------|
| 2/3 cup | 5 oz. |
| ½ cup | 4 oz. |
| 3 fl. oz. | 3 – 3 ½ oz. |
| ⅓ cup | 2 ½ -3 oz. |
| ¼ cup | 2-2 ½ oz. |
| 1 ½ fl. oz. | 1 ¾ oz. |
| 1 ⅓ fl. oz. | 1 ⅓ oz. |
| 1 fl. oz. | 1 oz. |
| 0.8 fl. oz. | 0.8 oz |
| ½ fl. oz. | ½ oz. |

## Temperature
<u>To convert Fahrenheit into Celsius:</u>

Subtract 32. Then multiply by 5/9.

*Example*: Convert 140°F to Celsius.
140-32=108
108x 5/9 = 60°C

<u>To convert Celsius to Fahrenheit:</u>

Multiply by 9/5. Then add 32.

*Example*: Convert 150°C to Fahrenheit.
150 x 9/5 = 270
270 + 32 = 302.

## Volume
1 fluid ounce = 29.57 milliliters
1 milliliter = 0.034 ounce
1 quart = 946 milliliters
1 liter equals 33.8 fluid ounces

## Weight
1 ounce = 28.35 grams
1 gram = 0.035 ounces
1 pound = 454 grams
1 kilogram = 2.2 pounds

## Length
1-inch = 25.4 millimeters
1 centimeter = 0.39 inch
1-meter = 39.4 inches

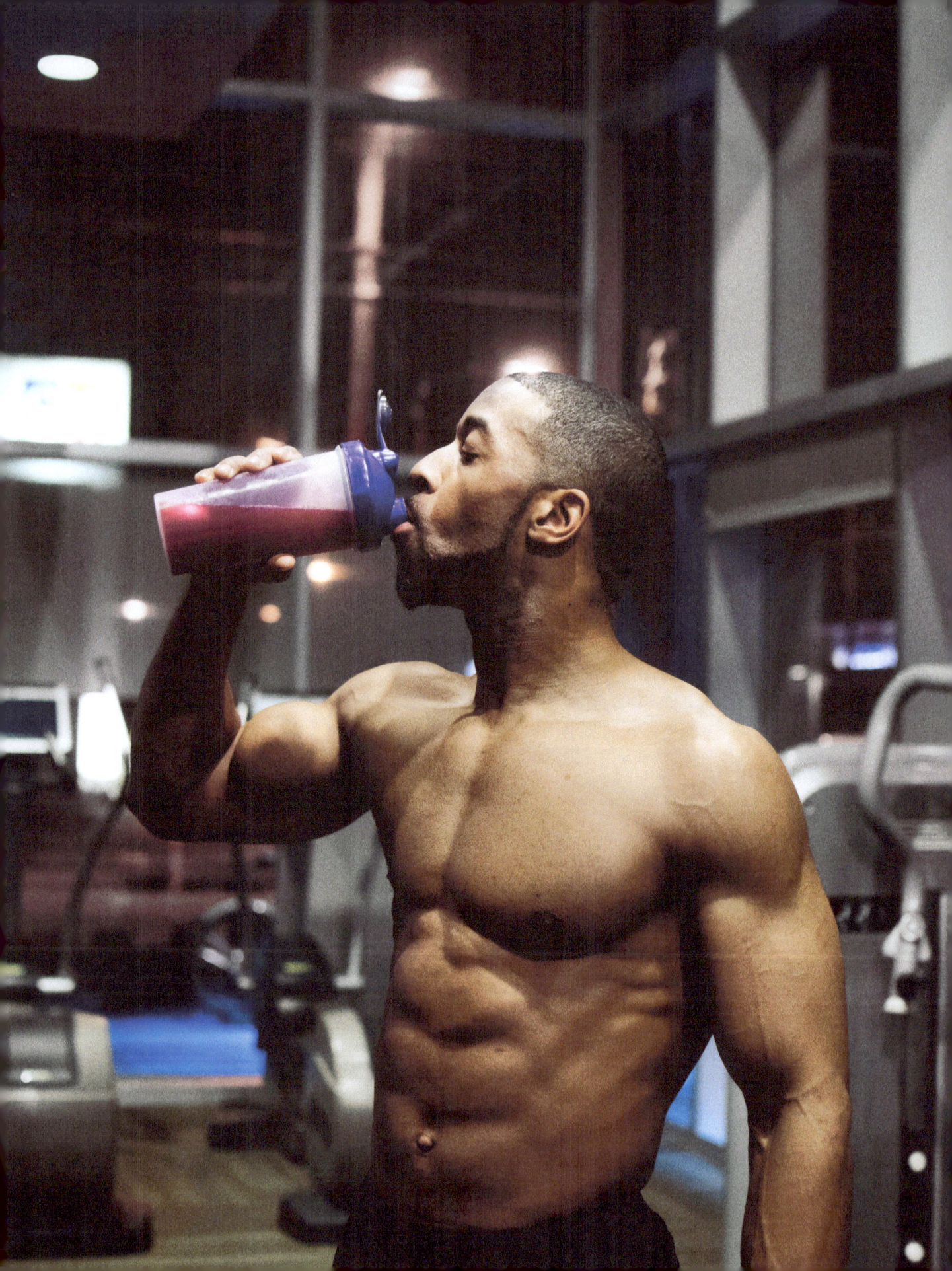

# JLUCAS NUTRITION TOP 10 SUPPLEMENT LIST FOR HEALTH & FITNESS

I've been taking supplements for over 20 years and started taking protein and creatine as a teenager. I was always known as the local supplement guru in high school. I told my track coach that I was taking creatine and he said "you'll burn up your liver!" He was just concerned for my safety, but after studying exercise physiology in college I learned that creatine isn't even metabolized by the liver and has one of the safest profiles of any supplement on the market.

Lots of people are concerned about the efficacy and safety of supplements and rightfully so. I am certainly a food first advocate, but I believe supplements can play a role in improving health and performance. Not all supplements are created equal which is why you should use references such as www.Labdoor.com, the NSF for Sport ® App http://www.nsfsport.com/news-resources/certified-for-sport-app.php, Informed Choice http://informed-choice.org/ and www.examine.com to do your research on what name brands are credible. The other issue you could run into when it comes to the efficacy and safety of supplements is how much of it you should take and the indications for use. Too much of anything may be harmful, so you want to stick to the suggested serving sizes.

With my long term experience taking supplements I have rarely experienced any side effects or illness because I have done my research, aimed to choose credible products, eat a healthy diet with good exercise habits and did not abuse the suggested serving sizes.

There are some individuals that are certainly skeptics of supplements and believe that it has no added benefits on health or performance but I can say that for me taking supplements has been fun, tasty and exuberant! It is a personal choice if you want to take and invest in supplements, but there is never a guarantee that it will give you the results you seek. At the end of the day, hard work and dedication will trump any magic bullet! Supplements generally are incredibly interesting to me to think about how an isolated nutrient or a combination of ingredients could have a synergistic effect on your body to produce a specific metabolic or physiological advantage. Use my top ten supplement guide as a rubric to decide upon what to take, how to take it and what potential benefit it may offer for your health and fitness!

This guide is intended to be used for educational and information purposes only. I am not advocating nutritional supplementation over proper medical advice or treatment. If using any pharmaceuticals or drugs given to you by a doctor or received with a prescription, you must consult with the doctor in question or an equally qualified health care professional prior to using any nutritional supplementation. If undergoing medical therapies, then consult with your respective therapist or health care professional about possible interactions between your treatment, any pharmaceuticals or drugs being given, and possible nutritional supplements or practices suggested by JLucas Nutrition.

# Chart Guide

| Supplement | What it is? | Potential benefit | How to take it | Health concerns/ safety |
|---|---|---|---|---|
| Branched Chain Amino Acids (BCAAs) | BCAAs are three amino acids leucine, isoleucine & valine with similar structures that beneficially influence the muscles. They can be found in protein rich foods, such as eggs or meat. They are the main energy producing amino acids for the skeletal muscles. | Decrease fatigue during exercise, spare muscle glycogen, increase time to exhaustion during endurance exercise, stimulate muscle protein synthesis | Take between meals, during fasting or during exercise. Aim for a product that provides 2g of leucine for every 1g of isoleucine & valine for a 2:1:1 ratio. Leucine is the main amino acid to stimulate muscle protein synthesis. | The tolerable upper limit is set at 500mg/ kg bodyweight (about 35g daily for average weight males). The average daily serving from supplements would be approximately 4g. |
| Caffeine also known as: Coffee extract, Tea extract, 1,3,7-Trimethylxanthine, Liquid crack | Caffeine is a stimulatory anti-sleep compound extracted from coffee beans. Caffeine's main mechanism concerns antagonizing adenosine receptors. Adenosine causes sedation and relaxation when it acts upon its receptors, located in the brain. Caffeine prevents this action and causes alertness and wakefulness. Caffeine is naturally present in coffee, tea, cocoa, guarana, and yerba mate, but it is also frequently added to sodas, energy drinks, and weight loss supplements. | Caffeine is a powerful stimulant, and it can be used to improve mental stimulation, physical strength and endurance. Some other potential benefits of caffeine include fat burning, and appetite suppression | Caffeine dosages should be tailored to individuals. If you are new to caffeine supplements, start with a 100mg dose. Typically, 200mg of caffeine is used for fat-burning supplementation, while acute strength increases occur at higher doses, 500mg and above. Caffeine can be supplemented through popular beverages, like Coffee, Tea and Energy Drinks, but it can also be taken in a pill form. Many of caffeine's effects, including fat burning, strength benefits, and euphoria, are subject to tolerance, and may not occur in people used to caffeine, no matter how large the dose is. | Caffeine is highly stimulatory and a systemic vasoconstrictor. Caution should be exerted if one is either not used to caffeine ingestion or currently has high blood pressure.

Caffeine should not be used as a supplement in those with cardiac impairments without prior consultation of one's doctor.

Caffeine can also have an effect on ones quality of sleep; while you may be able to fall asleep, it will be of inferior quality. |

| Supplement | What it is? | Potential benefit | How to take it | Health concerns/ safety |
|---|---|---|---|---|
| Casein – The 'nighttime' protein | Out of the 'curds and the whey' of milk, Casein protein is the curds. A dietary protein source with gel-forming capabilities, it is touted to be slowly absorbed in part due to slowing intestinal motility and gel-forming like fiber; adding water makes pudding. Found in milk based foods such as Greek Yogurt and cottage cheese. | Supports protein needs, helps build and preserve muscle mass over an extended period of time. Known as the slow digesting protein, providing a continuous influx of amino acids to the skeletal muscle. May help to improve body composition, support weight gain and performance. | Use as a meal replacement or snack between spaced-out meals to reduce hunger and overeating. Take 30-40g of casein protein before bed for increased muscle protein synthesis overnight without influencing the body's ability to breakdown fat. Use to cook with or prepare desserts (such as cheesecake) to enhance their protein content. | Avoid with any milk intolerances or milk allergies. |
| Creatine also known as: a-methylguan-idinoacetic acid, creatine mono-hydrate, creatine 2-oxopropanoate | Creatine is a molecule in an energy system (creatine phosphate) that can rapidly produce energy (ATP) to support cellular function. A pound of uncooked beef and salmon provide 1-2g of creatine. Creatine is made from the amino acids arginine, glycin and methionine from the liver and pancreas. | Creatine increases skeletal muscle creatine content for improved athletic performance in repeated bouts of maximal and endur-ance spriting. It also increases muscle mass, force, and power output with resistance training. | To realize the benefits of creatine quickly load with approximately 20-25g/ day in 4-5 split, 5g doses for 5-7 days. Otherwise to receive benefits overtime, take 5g of creatine per day indefinitely. Those with large muscle mass may consider 10g per day. Try taking 5g of creatine before and after exercise with a snack, meal or protein shake.  Cre-atine monohydrate is the cheapest and most effective. | Stomach cramping can occur when cre-atine is supplemented without sufficient water. Diarrhea and nausea can occur when too much cre-atine is supplemented at once, in which case doses should be spread out through-out the day and taken with meals. |

| Supplement | What it is? | Potential benefit | How to take it | Health concerns/ safety |
| --- | --- | --- | --- | --- |
| Fish oil - also known as: Eicos-apentaenoic acid (EPA), docosa-hexaenoic acid (DHA), Omega-3 fatty acids, Omega-3, Omega 3, N-3 fatty acids. | Fish oil contains omega three fatty acids EPA and DHA which are omega 3 fatty acids found in fish, animal products and phytoplankton. EPA and DHA are essential fatty acids which means they must be obtained from the diet to produce its physiological functions and to obtain the benefits associated with ingestion. | Adequate intake of fish oils are associated with healthier blood vessels, lower lipid count (LDLs) and reduced risk for plaque buildup (lowers triglycerides). Fish oil is also known to reduce inflammation and may be associated with reducing depression, slight memory improvements, blood pressure, risk for diabetes and cancers. | Benefits may occur over weeks of supplementation. A proper ratio of omega 3:6 EPA to DHA. For general health, 250mg is the minimum dose. The American Heart Association recommends 1g daily. If the goal of supplementation is to reduce soreness, a 6g dose, spread over the course of a day, will be effective. Fish oil is a general health supplement, and is taken as a source of omega-3 fats. It is not needed if one eats enough fatty fish (see "Omega-3 Fatty Acid Rich Foods" section) | To minimize the "fish burp" taste, take fish oil with meals, also you can consider freezing the fish oil pills and taking them frozen. Fish oil can reduce blood clotting and should be supplemented with caution if blood-thinning medications, asprin, warfarin or clopidogrel are already present in the body. |
| HMB – also known as Hydroxy-MethylButyrate, beta-hydroxy-beta-methylbutyrate | HMB is an active metabolite of Leucine that reduces muscle protein breakdown. It appears to have an anticatabolic role for muscle, but fails to be more effective than its parent amino acid for inducingmuscle protein synthesis. | HMB is associated with enhancing recovery, supporting lean body mass, strength, power and aerobic performance. Reduce muscle breakdown/ damage in aging muscle tissue or disease states such as HIV or cancer, may help reduce fat mass in combination with exercise | HMB is commercially available in powder or capsular form as mono-hydrated calcium salt (HMB-Ca) or in free acid form as HMB-free acid (HMB-FA). The most optimal dose may be 3g of HMB/d or 38mg/kg HMB daily. Consume 3g HMB at least 60 min prior to exercise. In order to optimize on HMB's chronic effects, take 1g HMB three times per day, a minimum of two weeks prior to a potentially damaging skeletal muscle event. | HMB is safe in both young and old populations. |
| Probiotics, Prebiotics, & Digestive Enzymes | | | | |

| Supplement | What it is? | Potential benefit | How to take it | Health concerns/ safety |
|---|---|---|---|---|
| Psyllium Husk Also known as: Psyllium Husk, Psyllium Fiber, Metamucil (brand name), ispaghula, plantago psyllium, plantago ovata, plantago | Psyllium (usually as husk or powder) is a soluble, gel forming fiber derived from the plant Plantago psyllium that is able to bind to fatty acids and cholesterol from the diet; it can increase fecal moisture and weight. | May help to significantly reduce appetite, may not reduce overall food intake; May help to reduce cholesterol in persons with high cholesterol; may help to reduce blood glucose in persons with high blood glucose; may help to reduce carbohydrate absorption; | Mix at least 200mL of water or more with 5g of psyllium with each meal. | Acute doses of up to 30g appear to be well tolerated assuming enough water (in these instances, around 500mL or so) are also coingested. Not associated with excess flatulence. You may want to consider taken separately from minerals like iron and calcium. Psyllium should be taken with water acutely, and placement of psyllium powder or husk into the mouth without water may result in sapping of saliva and subsequent choking. |
| Whey Protein - also known as: whey, whey concentrate, whey isolate, whey hydrolysate, hydrolyzed whey | Whey is a component of Milk Protein, with the other being casein. Whey may be healthier than other forms of protein. The benefits of whey are due to the protein itself, while casein may be a better muscle builder. | May have a minor effect on reducing fat mass when following a low calorie diet. May help to meet protein needs and promote lean body mass (muscle) when combined with a resistance exercise program. | Whey is used as a protein supplement. It is very useful for hitting targeted daily protein goals. Whey is absorbed faster than other forms of protein, which means it also increases muscle protein synthesis. | Whey is a food supplement, although products could be contaminated or spiked with banned substances or heavy metals. Use the references above to choose a high quality product. |

| Supplement | What it is? | Potential benefit | How to take it | Health concerns/ safety |
|---|---|---|---|---|
| Vitamin D - also known as: Cholecalciferol (Vitamin D3), Ergocalciferol (Vitamin D2) | Vitamin D is a fat-soluble, essential vitamin known as the sunlight vitamin, since it is synthesized in the skin when exposed to the sun's radiation. It provides benefits for bone structure support, mood state, and much more. Vitamin D is also found naturally in fish and eggs. It is also added to dairy products. | It is reported that there is a vitamin D receptor on every cell of the body, thus having an adequate vitamin D status may be beneficial for several functions: Reduce risk for falls in the elderly, reduce cardiovascular disease risk, reduce colorectal cancer risk, reduce bone fracture risk | Most people do not have an optimal level of vitamin D, therefore, supplementation is encouraged if optimal levels are not present in the body. The recommended daily allowance for Vitamin D is currently set at 400-800IU/day, but this is too low for adults. The safe upper limit in the United States is 2,000IU/day, while in Canada it is 4,000IU/day. Research suggests that the true safe upper limit is 10,000IU/day. For moderate supplementation, a 1,000-2,000IU dose of vitamin D3 is sufficient to meet the needs of most of the population. This is the lowest effective dose range. Higher doses, based on body weight, are in the range of 20-80IU/kg daily. Vitamin D3 supplementation (cholecalciferol) is recommended over D2 supplementation (ergocalciferol), since D3 is used more effectively in the body. Vitamin D should be taken daily, with meals or a source of fat, like Fish Oil | Acute doses of up to 30g appear to be well tolerated assuming enough water (in these instances, around 500mL or so) are also coingested. Not associated with excess flatulence. You may want to consider taken separately from minerals like iron and calcium. Psyllium should be taken with water acutely, and placement of psyllium powder or husk into the mouth without water may result in sapping of saliva and subsequent choking.

Toxicity from vitamin D is mediated by altering calcium metabolism, which is potentially lethal. Doses should not exceed 10,000IU daily unless supervised by a medical professional. |

JLucas Nutrition Top Ten Supplement List for Health & Fitness Adapted from: Examine.com Supplement-Goals Reference Guide: June 3, 2018

# JLUCAS NUTRITION MEAL PLANS FOR HEALTH & FITNESS

If you are looking for a specific meal plan and want more great meal plans to follow besides the "Rapper's Delight" meal plan which is based upon the Hip Hop Recipe Book for Health and Fitness then go to my website: jlucasnutrition.com You will find meal plans for Weight Loss & Wellness https://jlucasnutrition.com/weight-loss-wellness/ and for Muscle Building & Sports Performance https://jlucasnutrition.com/muscle-building-sports-performance/. I also offer Customized Meal Plans https://jlucasnutrition.com/customized-meal-plans/ for a more "tailor" fit for your goals and needs. See more specifics on the meal plans I offer below:

## Weight Loss & Wellness Meal Plans

Have you been struggling with weight loss? Tried many remedies to no avail? JLucas Nutrition offers several realistic weight loss approaches to help you to achieve long-term weight loss success. Choose from one of the following weight loss meal plan options to begin weight loss, that stays off! 7-Day Mediterranean Meal Plan, 28 day Low Cholesterol Diet Meal Plan, 28 day "True Paleo Auto Immune" Meal Plan, 28 day  Weight Loss Meal Plan, 28-Day Weight Loss Plan for Men, 28 day Weight Loss Plan for Women, 28 day True Paleo FODMAP Meal Plan, 28 day True Paleo Pescatarian Meal Plan, 7 day Rapper's Delight Meal Plan

Stay ahead of your health, uplift your wellness and reduce risk for disease with one of these weight loss and wellness meal plan options: Go to: https://jlucasnutrition.com/weight-loss-wellness/ for a list of all Weight Loss & Wellness Meal Plans.

**7 DAY MEDITERRANEAN MEAL PLAN**

The Mediterranean meal plan is the perfect if you are looking for a heart-healthy eating plan. This meal plan incorporates the basics of healthy eating in addition to those eating habits traditionally found in the countries surrounding the Mediterranean. You will find that this meal plan is rich in fruits and vegetables, whole grains and other healthy starches such as legumes and beans. In addition, it contains generous amounts of healthy fats, especially the heart healthy monounsaturated fats, by including foods such as olive oil, fish, nuts and seeds and limiting poultry and red meats. A 50% carbohydrate, 20% protein, 30% fat meal plan. Start following the 7 day Mediterranean Meal Plan by clicking here:

## 28 DAY LOW CHOLESTEROL MEAL PLAN
The average American diet consists of 510 mg of dietary cholesterol per day. The Low Cholesterol meal plan provides less than 120 mg of cholesterol per day. The meal plan contains plenty of fiber-rich foods including grains and vegetables which will help in lowering LDL levels (bad cholesterol) and triglycerides. By combining a regular exercise program with this meal plan you can raise HDL (good cholesterol) levels and prevent future health problems. The primary source of proteins comes from fish and poultry. Meals are distributed between 5 to 6 meals each day to boost metabolism. A 65% carbohydrates, 20% protein, 15% fat meal plan. Start following the 28 day Low Cholesterol Meal Plan by clicking here:

## 28 DAY "TRUE PALEO AUTO IMMUNE" MEAL PLAN
There are a few extra foods, like nightshade plants, nuts, seeds and egg whites, in addition to the standard Paleo diet, that one needs to avoid if dealing with an autoimmune issue. Here's an easy way to get the hang of your new healthy eating plan to help get you as healthy as you can be, and focus on everything you can eat, rather than feeling like you're in food jail! A 25% carbohydrate, 25% protein, 50% fat meal plan. Start following the 28 day "True Paleo Auto Immune" Meal Plan by clicking here:

## 28 DAY WEIGHT LOSS MEAL PLAN
The Weight Loss meal plan has been designed to yield fast results by combining the cleanest (low in fats), highest quality foods possible distributed between 5 to 6 meals each day to boost metabolism. Protein sources are provided by lean meats such as chicken, turkey and fish. This meal plan may be somewhat limited in variety but has been clinically proven to shed weight quickly when combined with a regular exercise routine consisting of cardiovascular exercises to burn calories and resistance exercises to maintain muscle tissue. A 50% carbohydrate, 35% protein, 15% fat meal plan. Start following the 28 day Weight Loss Meal Plan by clicking here:

## 28-DAY WEIGHT LOSS PLAN FOR MEN
The Weight Loss meal plan is very popular amongst male and female fitness enthusiasts to burn fat and maintain muscle. The Weight Loss meal plan has been designed to yield fast results by combining the cleanest (low in fats),

highest quality foods possible distributed between 5 to 6 meals each day to boost metabolism. Protein sources are provided by lean meats such as chicken, turkey and fish. This meal plan has been clinically proven to shed weight quickly when combined with a regular exercise routine consisting of cardiovascular exercises to burn calories and resistance exercises to maintain muscle tissue. A 45% carbohydrate, 25% protein, 30% fat meal plan. Start following the 28-Day Weight Loss Plan for Men by clicking here:

## 28 DAY WEIGHT LOSS PLAN FOR WOMEN
The Weight Loss meal plan is very popular amongst male and female fitness enthusiasts to burn fat and maintain muscle. The Weight Loss meal plan has been designed to yield fast results by combining the cleanest (low in fats), highest quality foods possible distributed between 5 to 6 meals each day to boost metabolism. Protein sources are provided by lean meats such as chicken, turkey and fish. This meal plan has been clinically proven to shed weight quickly when combined with a regular exercise routine consisting of cardiovascular exercises to burn calories and resistance exercises to maintain muscle tissue. A 45% carbohydrate, 25% protein, 30% fat meal plan. Start following the 28 day Weight Loss Plan for Women by clicking here:

## 28 DAY TRUE PALEO FODMAP MEAL PLAN
There are a few extra foods, in addition to the standard Paleo diet, that one needs to avoid if following a low FODMAP diet. Here's an easy way to get the hang of your new healthy eating plan to help get you as healthy as you can be and put an end to GI distress from eating certain foods. A 20% carbohydrate, 30% protein, 50% fat meal plan. Start following the 28 day True Paleo FODMAP Meal Plan by clicking here: https://jlucasnutrition.com/my-account/membership-checkout/?level=4

## 28 DAY TRUE PALEO PESCATARIAN MEAL PLAN
Interested in Paleo but not keen on eating meat or poultry? Not a problem. We can rely on a variety of wild fish to provide high quality protein without compromising nutrition. A 25% carbohydrate, 25% protein, 50% fat meal plan. Start following the 28 day True Paleo Pescatarian Meal Plan by clicking here:

## 7 DAY RAPPER'S DELIGHT MEAL PLAN
A hip-hop themed, healthy twist to common breakfast, lunch and dinner dishes for health and fitness! Provides a balanced ratio of protein, fat and carbohydrates to support lean body mass, muscle and to support fat loss. Comes with 21 hip-hop themed recipes inspired by one of your favorite hip hop artist. Start following the Rapper's Delight meal plan today to start seeing Simple, Real, Results! Based upon The Hip Hop Recipe Book for Health and Fitness! Start following the Rapper's Delight Meal Plan by clicking here:

# Muscle Building & Sports Performance Meal Plans

Looking to build muscle mass, gain weight, tone-up or enhance exercise performance? Choose from one of the following meal plan options to help meet your muscle building and sports performance goals: Muscle builder, Mass Builder/ Weight Gain, Lean and Tone, Paleo Strength Training or Paleo Triathlete, Lean Vegetarian Lifestyle Meal Plan, Lean for Speed Meal Plan

### 7 DAY MUSCLE BUILDER MEAL PLAN

Designed with the hard-gainer in mind. The Muscle Builder meal plan provides meal plans and foods that yield higher carbohydrates and slightly higher fat to pack on the pounds where fast weight gain is desired. This meal plan has been designed to work in conjunction with a regular weight training program to stimulate muscle tissue growth. Meal replacement shakes are required for snack times to boost daily calories and provide convenience over preparing foods. The animal protein sources for these meal plans come from chicken, turkey, fish and red meats. A 50% carbohydrate, 30%, protein, 20% fat meal plan. Start following the 7 day Muscle builder Meal Plan by clicking here:

### 7 DAY MASS BUILDER/ WEIGHT GAIN MEAL PLAN

Designed with the hard-gainer in mind. The Muscle Builder meal plan provides meal plans and foods that yield higher carbohydrates and slightly higher fat to pack on the pounds where fast weight gain is desired. This meal plan has been designed to work in conjunction with a regular weight training program to stimulate muscle tissue growth. Meal replacement shakes are required for snack times to boost daily calories and provide convenience over preparing foods. The animal protein sources for these meal plans come from chicken, turkey, fish and red meats. A 50% carbohydrate, 30%, protein, 20% fat meal plan. Start following the 7 day Mass Builder/ Weight Gain Meal Plan by clicking here: https://jlucasnutrition.com/my-account/membership-checkout/?level=5

### 7 DAY LEAN AND TONE PHYSIQUE MEAL PLAN

The Lean and Tone Physique meal plans combine higher protein, lower fat and higher daily calories for the average person wanting to shed body fat, entry level or experienced bodybuilder or fitness competitor. This meal plan has been designed using the cleanest (low in fats), highest quality foods possible distributed between 5 to 6 meals each day to maintain a high metabolism. Protein sources are provided by lean meats such as chicken, turkey, fish and generic protein shakes. This meal plan may be somewhat limited in variety but has been clinically proven to maintain or increase lean muscle tissue. A 50% carbohydrate, 35% protein, 15% fat meal plan. Start following the 7 day Lean and Tone Physique Meal Plan by clicking here:

## 28 DAY PALEO STRENGTH TRAINING OR PALEO TRIATHLETE MEAL PLAN

A 4 week paleo-based nutritional plan for multisport and/or endurance athletes. Perfect to use in conjunction with your training to optimize on athletic performance. A 50% carbohydrate, 30% protein, 20% fat meal plan. Start following the 28 day Paleo Strength Training or Paleo Triathlete Meal Plan by clicking here:

## 7 DAY LEAN VEGETARIAN LIFESTYLE MEAL PLAN

The Low Fat Vegetarian template provides 7 days of meal plans each consisting of 5-6 meals each day. The macronutrient ratios average 65% carbohydrates, 15% protein and 20% fat for the seven day period. Protein sources are provided by tofu and soy products, beans, peanuts and some diary in the form of cheese and milk (no eggs). This template may be somewhat limited in variety but has been clinically proven to shed weight quickly when combined with a regular exercise routine consisting of cardiovascular exercises to burn calories. A 65% Carbohydrate, 15%, Protein, 20% Fat meal plan. Start following the Lean Vegetarian Lifestyle Meal Plan by clicking here:

## 7 DAY LEAN FOR SPEED MEAL PLAN

Are you a track athlete or football player or perhaps looking to optimize on your physique or athletic performance? Check out this Lean for Speed 7 day diet plan, which lays out the foods you need for each meal for the development of a lean for speed physique. Start following the Lean for Speed Meal Plan by clicking here:

## 28 DAY PALEO STRENGTH TRAINING

Advice on what is Paleo and what is not can vary greatly from one gym affiliate to the next. This plan spells it out for you, completely in keeping with a True Paleo approach! This True Paleo nutritional plan for the strength is perfect to use in conjunction with your current training schedule. A 4 week paleo-based nutritional plan for multisport and/or endurance athletes. Perfect to use in conjunction with your training regimen. A 25% carbohydrate, 30% protein, 45% fat meal plan. Start following the Paleo Strength Training by clicking here:

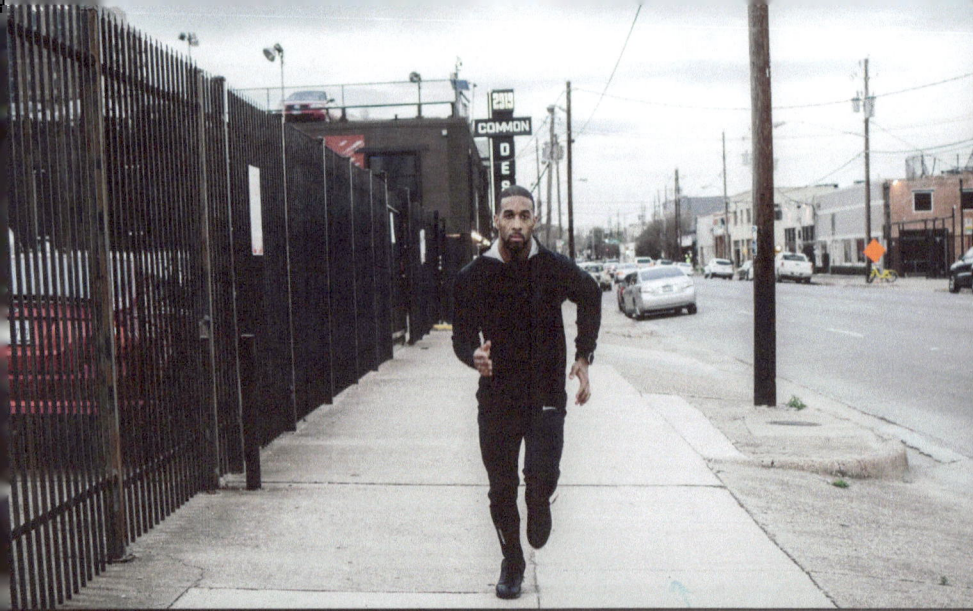

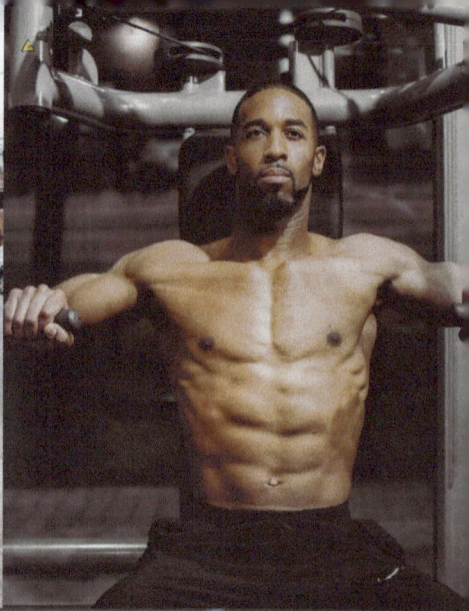

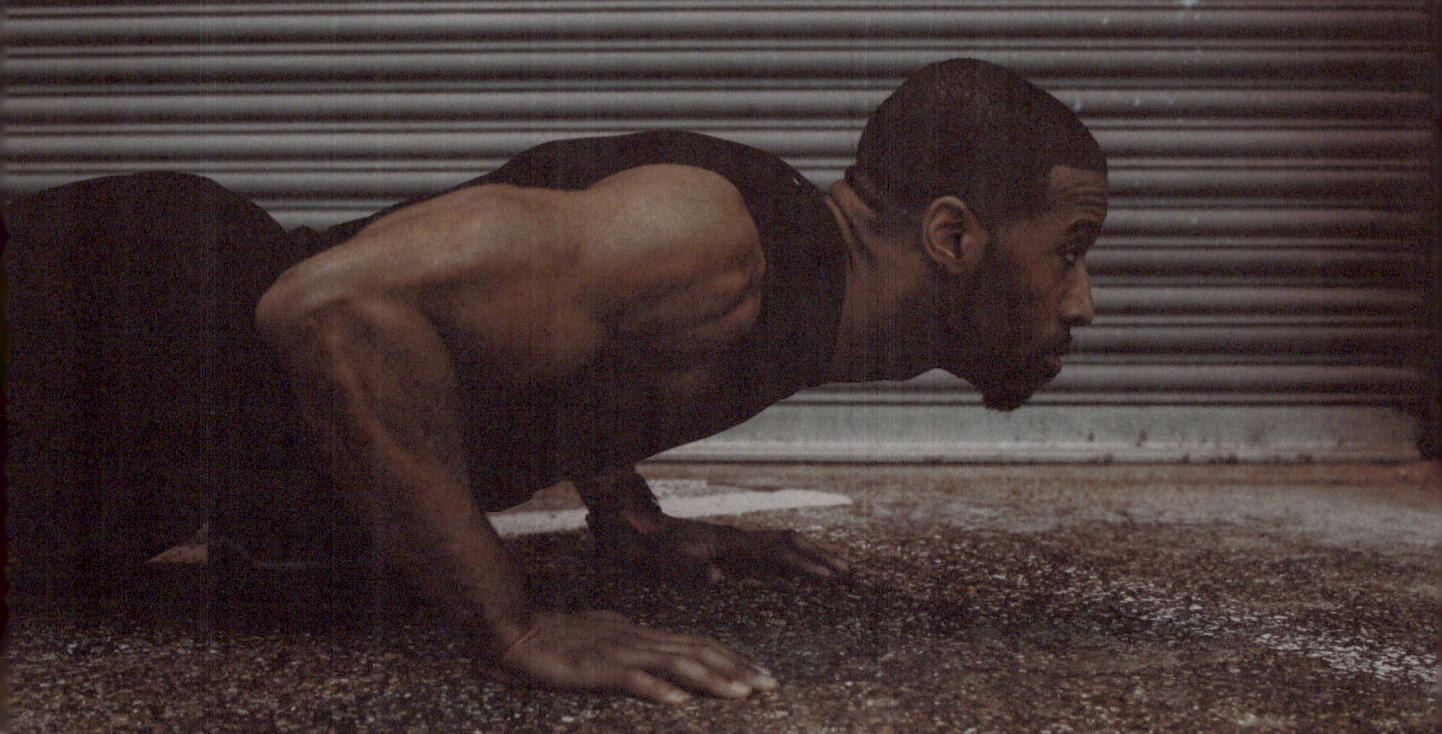

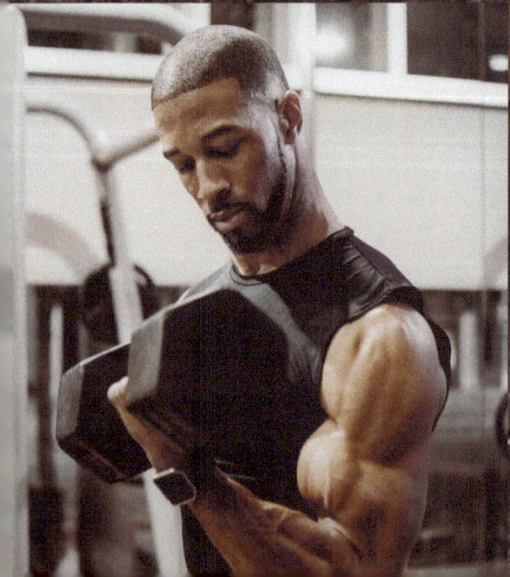

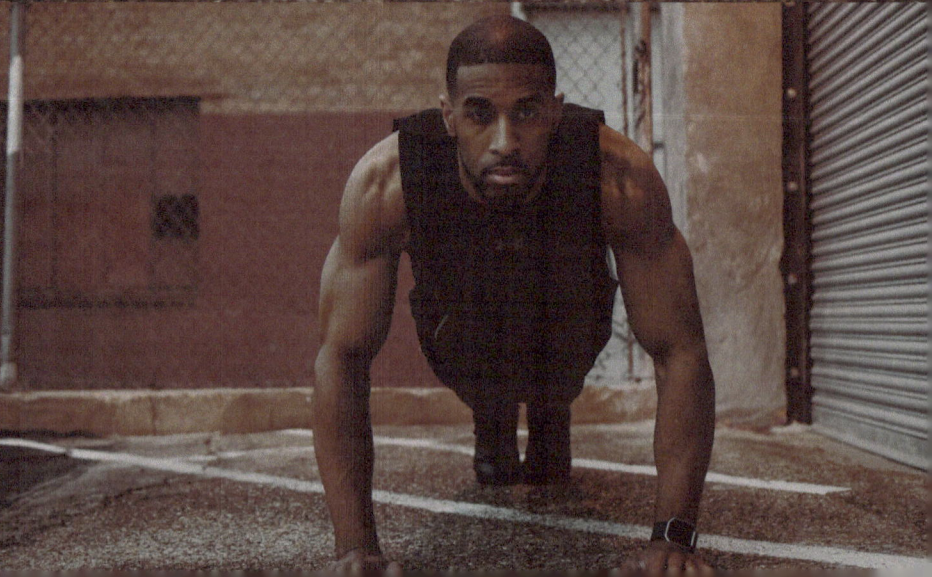

# JLUCAS NUTRITION TOP 10 EXERCISE TIPS FOR HEALTH & FITNESS

There are a lot fitness guru's with many different philosophies on the best exercises to get in shape. I am not here to tell you that my tips are the best to help you meet your fitness goals, but I am here to provide you with some sound advice based on some evidence and real world experience that I have. I have been working out in gyms since I was 12 and I certainly don't know everything, but I have picked up a few tips from gym rats, coaches, teammates and some exercise physiology courses. I can guarantee you with discipline and consistency you will improve your health and fitness. Here are my top 10 exercise tips for health & fitness, choose the ones that apply best for your needs:

**1.** **THE MORE YOU MOVE, THE MORE YOU LOSE!** — The gym might not be for everyone. You don't have to get in the gym to get in shape, but you should find something fun that will get you moving to keep you from gaining weight or to help you lose weight if that is your goal. Dancing, tennis, swimming, walking, find something that you enjoy doing to optimize on your physical activity and daily movement.

**2.** **KEEP IT NEAT!** — Make a mess, don't fret, keep cleaning and keeping it neat around the house. This will keep your waist line nice and neat! Any spontaneous movement such as tapping your feet while seated, taking the stairs, fidgeting and not sitting still can contribute to what's known as Non Exercising Activity Thermogenesis (NEAT). This small increase in physical activity can play an incremental role in the number of calories your burn per day. NEAT can be a critical component in how we maintain our body weight and could help to support a weight loss or fat loss effort. In other words NEAT can help you become more shredded! So keep your feet moving with NEAT!

**3.** **INCREASE THE INTENSITY!** — When I think of intensity I am referring to the amount of effort or force that you put into something. Think about the amount of intensity you put into anything. Usually when we go about accomplishing something and put a high amount of intensity then we come out with phenomenal results. This is where your intensity for exercise comes into play. Especially when we are talking about cardio. Do you feel like you will lose more weight and get into better shape walking, jogging or sprinting as hard and fast as you can? This is why Olympic sprinters have some of the most phenomenal bodies in the world. The greater the intensity the more you stimulate adrenaline, which then releases a hormone called hormone sensitive lipase which breaks fat down. High intensity exercise, particularly causes the greatest amount of fat breakdown from the mid-section (abdominals). I recommend doing cycle sprints for 30-60 seconds on the treadmill or stationary bike with a 1-2 minute rest in between each set. Aim for 4-10 sets of each set of sprints. I would incorporate these high intensity interval training (HIIT) routines twice per week approximately three days apart. Long-term slow jogging can lead to weight loss as well, but at the expense of lean body mass or muscle. Perhaps include a lower intensity exercise such as walking, jogging, swimming, elliptical or stair master for 30-60 minutes; 1-2 times per week may be helpful for long-term fat loss, but if your looking to lose weight faster while staying lean then HIIT is the way to go. Stick to HIIT if you want to burn body fat, increase your metabolism, preserve muscle mass and get shredded.

**4.** **TURN UP THE VOLUME!** — How many reps and sets do you put in at the gym? The total amount of work you put into your workout routine can lead to greater results. Aim for more reps and more sets! Lift moderately heavy, enough to do 8-15 reps, if you can't get to at least 8 reps on most exercises then I recommended lightening it up. I believe for men they become too concerned about not lifting heavy enough and for women they become concerned about lifting too much! I believe finding a happy medium is most appropriate for either gender.  Just remember the more exercise and reps you do the greater the total volume produced and the greater potential for body weight changes.

**5.** **BE DYNAMIC NOT STATIC!** — Many avid active individuals stretch or warm up before starting physical activity. I notice in the gym many people stretch before working out. This gives a sense of euphoria and it's what we are accustom to from gym class in grade school or organized sports. There is little to no supportive evidence suggesting that static stretching helps to prevent injury or improve athletic performance. However, if using dynamic stretching it can be more effective at improving athletic performance; increasing force production, power output, running speed, strength endurance and reaction time. Besides the performance benefits I love it because it gets your heart rate going, and helps you move more, so that you are burning more calories to support a lean and tone physique. Give yourself a solid ten minutes to  warm up with exercises such as push-ups, plyometrics, light jog to sprints, high knees, butt kicks, body weight lunges, squats & squat jumps; rotate the joints of the fingers, wrists, elbows, shoulders, neck, trunk, hips, ankles, feet and toes for better performance and overall calorie expenditure. Save static stretching for last, to cool down and relax the muscle fibers.

**6.** **KNOW WHAT REST IS BEST!** — Are you resting too much or too little between exercises? Your rest period between each exercise can play a big role in lean body mass gains and fat loss. A general rule of thumb is the heavier you lift the more rest you will need between sets. Typically 1-3 minutes is the average amount of time you should give yourself between each exercise set. If you are resting for too long you are probably not pushing yourself hard enough to get the most out of your workout. Burn out sets should always be saved for the last set of your workout; otherwise you may find yourself burnt out in the early stages of your workout, unable to lift more for extended periods of time. Larger muscle groups with power exercises such as bench press, squats, shoulder press, bent over rows with heavy loads require a three minute rest between sets to allow for the creatine phosphate energy system to replenish. If you are working smaller muscle groups such as biceps, triceps, doing lighter weights and higher reps then aim for one minute of rest between each set.

**7.** **LIGHTEN THE LOAD BEFORE YOU FOLD!** — If lifting heavy is your thing by all means. I am certainly not a power lifter and I stick to the weight that I am most comfortable with. If you're aiming to build strength and power then lifting heavier 4-5 sets of 5 reps or less may be best. When I played sports years ago I would adapt this principle, but nowadays I am working out for health and fitness and have found that very high reps work really well for me. I stick to 4-5 sets and between 10-20 reps for any one exercise. I start out with larger muscle groups and exercises that require a heavier load such as squats or bench press and I aim for 8 – 12 reps or more. As I progress through each exercise I am usually lightening the load and doing higher reps 10-20+ reps and several sets. You want to feel the burn, this is lactic acid. Lactic acid has been associated with stimulating muscle protein synthesis for more lean body mass gains.

**8.** **CHANGE THE RESISTANCE AND REMAIN PERSISTENT!** — Aim to use several different types of machines and weights to reach your fitness goals. Free weights, body weights, bands, selectorized machines are all great. You want to change your workout in some shape or form every 2-4 weeks. The floor surface, exercises, order of exercises, number of reps, sets and rest can all be ways by which you can change your workout routine to keep your muscles under tension and stress for greater results!

**9.** **KNOW YOUR CADENCE BEFORE YOU GET FADED!** — The cadence of your workout can also play a role in lean body mass gains. You have eccentric (the stretch, elongation of the muscle) and concentric (the push, shortening and contraction of the muscle). Many people focus on the concentric phase of the lift, but it is actually the eccentric phase of the lift where the most tension is placed on the muscle, this is where the muscle fibers are at its weakest point and little muscle fibers begin to tear with the load. I aim to move with a fast cadence on most lifts to get the most reps and sets as possible, while being under control to not cause injury. You want to cause some slight muscle damage on the eccentric phase as this is what causes the body to go into repair mode, to rebuild the muscle tissue for greater strength for the next lifts a.k.a. muscle gains and growth!

**10.** **BE A SUPER-GIANT IN THE GYM!** — Most active individuals will use a single exercise and perform that movement for 3-4 sets with rest. You can make this exercise more challenging by performing two (super set) or three or more (giant sets) within the same workout with little to no rest between each exercise. This is extremely difficult! I would recommend adding super sets and giant sets into your workout routine once you have trained for 1-3 months. Add supersets and giant sets to your last set of exercises. I can guarantee you that when you start to add super sets and giant sets into your workouts 2-3 times per week you will start to become more shredded (a.k.a. major fat loss). Just remember to put in the effort, intensity and mental focus to achieve your goal and stay persistent. Real body weight changes usually occur over a period of every 4 weeks, so don't expect magic! The only change you will see if based upon the work you put in, no short cuts!

# HIP-HOP NUTRITION VOLUME 1
## GROCERY LIST*

Get to the "bag" and improve your health with the Hip Hop Nutrition grocery list. BAG stands for **B**ehavioral **A**djustments for **G**reatness (coined by DJ Kelly G.). To be great you have to be willing to make adjustments to your behaviors. Invest in your health to get the most out of your wealth. #Healthiswealth

- [ ] Shredded Mild Cheddar, 8 Ounce
- [ ] Extra Virgin Olive Oil, 16.9 fl oz
- [ ] Tri-Color Pepper Strips, 14 Ounce (Frozen)
- [ ] Diced Onions, 10 oz
- [ ] 4 - Beefsteak Tomato, One Medium
- [ ] Egg Whites, 32.0 oz
- [ ] Carrot Chips, 16 oz bag
- [ ] Cucumber, Medium
- [ ] Chunk Light Tuna in Water, 5 Ounce Cans (Pack of 4)
- [ ] Hearts of Romaine, 3ct, 12 oz
- [ ] Craisins Reduced Sugar Dried Cranberries, 5 oz
- [ ] LITE Balsamic Vinaigrette Dressing, 16 fl oz
- [ ] Small Red Beans 15.5 oz
- [ ] 90% Lean Ground Beef, 1 lb
- [ ] Minced Garlic, 4.5 oz
- [ ] Sofrito, 12 oz
- [ ] Sazon 1.41 oz
- [ ] Cumin Seed, 1.48 oz
- [ ] Whole Grain Brown Rice, 10 ounce steamable bag
- [ ] Distilled White Vinegar, 16 Ounce
- [ ] Large, White Eggs, 1 Dozen
- [ ] Quick 1-Minute Oatmeal, Breakfast Cereal, 18oz Canister
- [ ] Almond Milk, Unsweetened Vanilla 64 oz
- [ ] Blueberries, 1 pint
- [ ] Walnut Halves and Pieces, 2.25 oz
- [ ] Boneless Skinless Chicken Breasts Individually Wrapped, 2 lb (Frozen)
- [ ] Baby Spinach, 5 oz
- [ ] Strawberries, 1 lb
- [ ] Navy Beans, 15 oz
- [ ] Cilantro, 1 oz (Bunch)
- [ ] Lean Ground Turkey, 16 oz
- [ ] Lime, One Medium
- [ ] Chili Powder, 4.5 oz
- [ ] Garlic Powder , 1.1 oz
- [ ] Steak Sauce, 10 oz
- [ ] Tomato Sauce, 8 oz
- [ ] 100% Whey Protein Powder, Vanilla, 2 lb
- [ ] Bananas, 1 bunch (min. 5 ct.)
- [ ] Psyllium Husk Whole Flakes, 12 oz
- [ ] Whole Strawberries, 32 oz, (Frozen)

- [ ] Berry Medley, 12 Ounce (Frozen)
- [ ] Asparagus, 1 bunch
- [ ] USDA Choice Beef Top Sirloin Steak, 8 oz
- [ ] Potatoes, 5 lb
- [ ] Steak Seasoning, 3.4 oz
- [ ] Honey Light Amber, 12 oz
- [ ] Almonds - Sliced, 8 oz
- [ ] Pure Canola Oil, 48 oz
- [ ] Coconut Flakes, 7 oz
- [ ] Ground Cinnamon, 1 oz
- [ ] Salmon Fillet, 12 oz, (Frozen)
- [ ] Sea Salt Grinder (Convenient & Adjustable), 2.12 oz
- [ ] Lemon, One Medium
- [ ] Lemon & Pepper Seasoning, 3.5 oz
- [ ] Mashed Cauliflower with Sea Salt, 12 oz (frozen)
- [ ] Roasted Sweet Potatoes, 16 oz Bag (Frozen)
- [ ] Frozen Broccoli Cuts, 10.8 ounce steamable bag
- [ ] Buttery Spread with Extra Virgin Olive Oil, 13 oz
- [ ] Whipped Cream, Original, 6.5 oz

- [ ] CÎROC French Vanilla, 1.75L
- [ ] Mandarin Oranges, 10.5 oz
- [ ] Pineapple Chunks in Juice, 8 oz
- [ ] Corn Flakes Cereal, 18 oz
- [ ] Peanut Butter Creamy, 16 oz
- [ ] Pinto Beans No Salt Added, 15.5 oz
- [ ] Italian Parsley (Flat Leaf), 1 Bunch
- [ ] Yellow Squash, 1.5 lb
- [ ] Zucchini Squash, 1.5 lb
- [ ] Lite Soy Sauce, Cruet, 5 oz
- [ ] Minced Ginger, 6.7 Oz
- [ ] Instant Grits, 12 ct
- [ ] Wild Sardines (skinless, boneless), 4.4 Ounce
- [ ] Boneless, Skinless Chicken Tenders, 0.88 lb
- [ ] Spaghetti Squash
- [ ] Fresh Wild Alaskan Cod, Longline caught, 1 lb
- [ ] Italian Salad, 10 oz
- [ ] Rice Krispies Cereal, 12 oz
- [ ] French Bread, 20 oz
- [ ] Sugar Free Syrup, 12 oz

*This grocery list is designed to provide enough food to feed a household of one for approximately one month.

# REFERENCES

Burd NA, Phillips SM. Protein and exercise. In Rosenbloom CA, Coleman EJ, eds. Sports Nutrition: A Practice Manual for Professionals, 5th ed. Chicago, IL: Academy of Nutrition and Dietetics; 2012:36-57

Caron M, et al. Long-term nutritional impact of sleeve gastrectomy . Surg Obes Relat Dis. (2017)

Calton JB. Prevalence of micronutrient deficiency in popular diet plans . J Int Soc Sports Nutr. (2010)

Castaño E, et al. Folate and Pregnancy, current concepts: It is required folic acid supplementation? . Rev Chil Pediatr. (2017)

Craig WJ. Health effects of vegan diets . Am J Clin Nutr. (2009)

Crider KS, Bailey LB, Berry RJ. Folic acid food fortification-its history, effect, concerns, and future directions . Nutrients. (2011)

Doherty, T.J. (2003) Invited review: aging and sarcopenia. Journal of Applied Physiology; 95:1717-1727.

Erin Gaffney-Stomberg, Karl L. Insogna, Nancy R. Rodriguez, and Jane E. Kerstetter, "Increasing Dietary Protein Requirements in Elderly People for Optimal Muscle and Bone Health," Journal of the American Geriatrics Society 47, no. 6 (2009): 1073-79. Doi:10.1111/j.1532-5415.2009.02285.x.

Harris E, et al. No effect of multivitamin supplementation on central blood pressure in healthy older people: A randomized controlled trial . Atherosclerosis. (2016)

Harris WS. Omega-3 fatty acids. In: Coates PM, Betz JM, Blackman MR, et al., eds. Encyclopedia of Dietary Supplements. 2nd ed. London and New York: Informa Healthcare; 2010:577-86.

Fielding, R.A., Vellas, B., Evans, W.J., Bhasin, S., Morley, J.E., Newman, A.B.,…Zamboni, M. (2011). Sarcopenia: an undiagnosed condition in older adults. Current consensus definition: prevalence, etiology, and consequences. International working group on sarcopenia. Journal of the American Medical Directors Association; 12, 249–256.

Filippi J, et al. Nutritional deficiencies in patients with Crohn's disease in remission . Inflamm Bowel Dis. (2006)

Guan B, et al. Nutritional Deficiencies in Chinese Patients Undergoing Gastric Bypass and Sleeve Gastrectomy: Prevalence and Predictors . Obes Surg. (2018)

Levine, JA. Non-exercise activity thermogenesis (NEAT). Clinical Endocrinology & Metabolism. December 2002, Vol. 16, Issue 4, Pages 679-702

Milne, A.C., Avenell, A., Potter, J. (2006). Meta-analysis: protein and energy supplementation in older people. Annals of Internal Medicine; 144:37-48.

Morley, J.E., Baumgartner, R.N., Roubenoff, R., Mayer, J. and Nair, K. S. (2001). Sarcopenia. The Journal of Laboratory and Clinical Medicine. 137, 231–243.

Nair, K.S. (2005). Aging muscle. American Journal of Clinical Nutrition; 81, 953–963

Nowson, Caryl, and Stella O'Connell. "Protein Requirements and Recommendations for Older People: A Review." Nutrients 7.8 (2015): 6874–6899. PMC. Web. 27 Aug. 2018.

Oliver D. Witard, Sarah R. Jackman, Arie K. Kies, Asker E. Jeukendrup, and Kevin D. Tipton, "Effect of Increased Dietary Protein on Tolerance to Intensified Training," Medicine and Science in Sports and Exercise 43, no. 4 (2011): 598-607. Doi: 10.1249/MSS.0b013e3181f684c9

Park S, Johnson M, Fischer JG. Vitamin and mineral supplements: barriers and challenges for older adults . J Nutr Elder. (2008)

Sawaya RA, et al. Vitamin, mineral, and drug absorption following bariatric surgery . Curr Drug Metab. (2012)

U.S. Department of Agriculture, Agricultural Research Service. USDA National Nutrient Database for Standard Reference, Release 28.Nutrient Data Laboratory Home Page, 2015

Vici G, et al. Gluten free diet and nutrient deficiencies: A review . Clin Nutr. (2016)

Zhang Q, et al. Effect of folic acid supplementation on preterm delivery and small for gestational age births: A systematic review and meta-analysis . Reprod Toxicol. (2017)